B. Deixonne F.-M. Lopez (Eds.)

Operative Ultrasonography

During Hepatobiliary and Pancreatic Surgery

With the Collaboration of
M. Dauzat, M. Makuuchi, J. Mouroux, A. Pissas
and B. Sigel

Foreword by H. Baumel

With 124 Figures

Springer-Verlag Berlin Heidelberg New York
London Paris Tokyo

BERNARD DEIXONNE, M. D.
Unit of Hepato-Biliary and Pancreatic Surgery
Department of Surgery, Hôpital Caremeau
30000 Nîmes, France

FRANCOIS-MICHEL LOPEZ, M. D.
Professor of Radiology
University of Montpellier-Nîmes
Department of Medical Imaging, Hôpital Caremeau
30000 Nîmes, France

Translated by
Jacqueline Simon

ISBN-13: 978-3-642-95524-2 e-ISBN-13: 978-3-642-95522-8
DOI: 10.1007/978-3-642-95522-8

Library of Congress Cataloging in Publication Data
Operative ultrasonography during hepatobiliary and pancreatic surgery.
Includes bibliographies and index. 1. Liver - Ultrasonic imaging. 2. Biliary tract - Ultrasonic imaging. 3. Pancreas - Ultrasonic imaging. 4. Operative ultrasonography.
I. Deixonne, B (Bernard) II. Lopex, F.-M. (Francois-Michel), 1946 - III. Dauzat, Michel. [DNLM: 1. Billary Tract Surgery. 2. Interoperative Care. 3. Liver - surgery. 4. Pancreas - surgery. 5. Ultrasonic Diagnosis. WI 770 O61]
RD546.064 1988 617'.55607543 88-12185
ISBN-13: 978-3-642-95524-2

Softcover reprint of the hardcover 1st edition 1988

Typesetting,: Appl, Wemding
2121/3145-543210

“La main voit” - *The hand sees*

Foreword

Surgery an essentially manual exercise in its early days, has progressively grown richer in complementary techniques helping the surgeon to perfect his movements and increase efficiency. This is particularly the case with digestive surgery, which has been thoroughly transformed by radiology, endoscopy and extemporaneous examinations effected during surgical intervention. Such methods make it possible for surgeons to develop subtle nuances in operative techniques and to specify indications more and more precisely. Ultrasonography must now be included among such techniques. It supplements them and can sometimes even replace them. For these reasons, this work devoted to the use of ultrasound by the surgeon during surgical intervention is of great interest.

Two general conditions had to be met before ultrasonography could be employed in abdominal surgery: the method and apparatus had to be adapted to its surgical utilization, and the surgeon had to adapt to a nonsurgical technique. The first condition has been fulfilled for all purposes. Intraoperative sonograms can be generated at a very high rate and are proving to be more and more useful. The miniaturization of probes permits their application almost everywhere with optimal results. Of course, the costs are still high, but one can expect them to decrease.

Surgeons can only be trained by persistent practice enabling them to become acquainted with a technique whose theoretical foundations may not have been taught to them. They must revise their knowledge of descriptive and topographic anatomy in order to acquire a new echoanatomic bi- or tridimensional concept essentially founded on the notion of sections.

It is therefore not surprising that the authors dedicated the first part of this book to a long and precise description of ultrasonography, including the theoretical bases of sonography and the semeiologic aspects of its applications in medicine. The other chapters of the book deal with operative ultrasonography applied to surgery of the liver, biliary tract, and pancreas.

Wisely, the authors adopted the same plan for each of these three organs: descriptions of the anatomy, the signs, and the sonographic features characterizing the different conditions of the organs. This organization is clear and also allows one to have an idea about the comparative value of the explorative method for each of the organs. In effect, the liver, a voluminous viscus whose deep zones often escape direct exploration, appears to be the prime object. A surgeon can only be acquainted with their intimate anatomy by means of a mental reconstruction based on the segmentation remarkably described by Couinaud. In the future, intraoperative ultrasonography of the liver will enable the surgeon to detect small lesions seated deep inside. The capability of ultrasound to detect systematically nonvisible metastases is essential. Furthermore, during exeresis, ultrasonography provides the surgeon a guide by furnishing a vascular chart of the liver without which the progression to the interior parenchyma would be blind and based only on theoretical knowledge.

The pancreas, because of its parenchymatous structure and deep location on the posterior abdominal wall, also appears to be a good target for intraoperative ultrasonography, especially when searching for small lesions, studying the excretory duct, and examining large peripancreatic vessels. In contrast, the method does not appear to be very useful in characterizing the nature of pancreatic masses and differentiating cancer from pancreatitis.

This technique does not seem to be applicable to the biliary ducts, while preoperative transparietal echography is of great interest for their exploration. During intervention, ductular opacification and choledocoscopy apparently prove to be more reliable, sonography here being a purely complementary technique.

As the authors say, intraoperative ultrasonography is really the eye prolonging the surgeon's hand, giving him a sixth sense which neither his vision nor his hand can compete with. To describe it, the collaboration of radiologist and surgeon in this book is very significant; it effectively provides an example of interpenetrating branches of knowledge in modern medicine.

The authors' vast experience enables the reader to perceive, all at the same time, the novelty of what is today, the incomparability of what will be tomorrow, and the indispensability of what may still lie in the future.

Nîmes, Spring 1988

HUGHES BAUMEL
Professor of Surgery

Table of Contents

Coauthors

DAUZAT, MICHEL, M. D.
Department of Medical Imaging, Hôpital Caremeau
30000 Nîmes, France

MAKUUCHI, MASATOSHI, M. D.
Department of Surgery, National Cancer Center Hospital
Tokyo, Japan 104

MOUROUX, JEROME, M. D.
Department of Surgery, Hôpital Caremeau
30000 Nîmes, France

PISSAS, ALEXANDRE, M. D.
Department of Surgery, Centre Hospitalier
30200 Bagnols-sur-Cèze, France

SIGEL, BERNARD, M. D.
Professor and Chairman, Department of Surgery
Medical College of Pennsylvania
Philadelphia, PA 19129
USA

1 Introduction

B. Deixonne, F.-M. Lopez

Intraoperative ultrasonography "extends" the eye and hand of the surgeon. It has practical applications in various fields such as neurosurgery, and vascular, urologic, gastrointestinal, and general surgery.

1.1 Stages of Intraoperative Ultrasonography

The development of intraoperative ultrasonography has followed that of transparietal sonography, and has been based upon technical developments.

The first attempts to use ultrasonography during surgical intervention were proposed in 1961, during the era of unidimensional sonography. The equipment now in use is exceptionally specialized, but can also be adapted to perform other functions. The aim is essentially the diagnosis and localization of calculi.

In 1961, Schlegel et al. [4] used sonography to localize renal calculi by means of a sterile probe. Hayashi et al., in 1962, reported some examples of the diagnosis of gallbladder stones by means of a special laparoscope carrying a probe [2]. The year after, Knight and Newel [3], in Great Britain, published a few reports of common bile duct exploration during surgery for stones in the gallbladder. In 1965, Eiseman et al. reported 46 intraoperative explorations of the biliary ducts using sonography. First, they used a normal probe, then they perfected a miniaturized probe for introduction into the common bile duct. They detected 18 stones of the common bile duct and noticed two false-positive and two false-negative results [1].

However, the attempts to use sonography remained isolated, and the technique was not as successful as had been predicted. The methods used stayed at a rudimentary stage, and no real effort was made to employ it in research, as too many surgeons had been discouraged by the extreme difficulty of analyzing the transmitted images. On the other hand, since 1978, with the arrival of a new generation of sonograms yielding real-time images (mode B), several teams have used the new equipment and perfected it.

In hepatobiliary and pancreatic surgery, the pioneers were Sigel in the United States, Lane in Australia, and Makuuchi in Japan. From the beginning of 1978, Sigel dedicated himself to this technique and improved the first probe for intraoperative use: a sterilizable sectorial scanning probe made of stainless steel. However, its cumbersome nature limited its use to biliary duct and pancreatic exploration. Some time later, the perfection attained by the Japanese manufacturers of linear scanning probes that were less cumbersome allowed exploration of the liver under excellent conditions. Nowadays, numerous manufacturers are proposing materials especially adapted to intraoperative ultrasonography, so that this explorative method is starting to become widely used.

1.2 Intraoperative Sonography in Gastrointestinal Surgery

Intraoperative sonography satisfies a wider range of interests than X-ray imaging. For technical reasons, it does not provide any information for orthopedic surgery. In the search for calculi and abnormalities of ductular systems such as the biliary ducts or excretory urinary ducts, its contribution is complementary to that of radiology with peroperative opacification.

Ultrasonography is much more interesting for exploration of vessels, which are directly visualized without any artifice, whereas vascular examination by X-ray requires complex and expensive appliances, which are difficult to use. Very rarely are operating rooms equipped with such appliances. It has an essential role in detecting, localizing, and checking the extension of parenchymatous lesions, especially when they are small and deep-seated. This explains the enthusiasm for it in neurosurgery, in which the opportunities for inspection and palpation are relatively limited. In gastrointestinal surgery, it is becoming more and more important in exploration and intraoperative examination because of the information it provides about biliary ducts, the liver, the pancreas, arteries and veins. In intraoperative biliary duct exploration, it is used alongside and as a complement to cholangiography and choledochoscopy, techniques which are currently widely employed by surgeons.

Vascular examination has been, and still is, limited to ileoportography. For practical reasons related to the equipment of the operating room, this examination is occasionally used, essentially to assess the integrity of the mesentericoportal venous axis. This vascular exploration is now easy, thanks to sonography which, furthermore, can be used to explore the whole of the perilesional vascular system, both arterial or venous, with precision.

The pancreas has the advantages of being relatively small, accessible to palpation, and traversed by the common bile duct and principal pancreatic duct. Here again, opacification of these ductal structures yields a certain amount of information, which is often only an indirect indication of a pathological process. Sonography is a great help, as much for the information it provides about the parenchyma as for the facilitation of pancreatic duct catheterization when opacification of the duct seems to be necessary, or for taking samples of pancreatic juice.

The liver remains poor in terms of the range of complementary intraoperative explorations that can be performed. There are practically none. Besides inspection and palpation - the latter being difficult because of the thickness of the intervening tissues - we cannot rely on the information provided by cholangiography or ileoportography. Intraoperative ultrasonography can provide information about the hepatic parenchyma that radiology is unable to give.

Finally, exploration of the accessory glands, which is mainly a concern of tumoral pathology, has been limited, often to what can be seen or felt. However, the important thing is to discover what we do not see spontaneously or what is not palpable. Prior to the advent of sonography, no intraoperative examination easily permitted visualization of parenchymatous structures and their vascularization. One can easily conceive of the tremendous interest that this technique offers, in addition to its advantages of being innocuous, noninvasive and easy to carry out. Nonetheless, this technique requires, on the part of the surgeon, a rather long training period. He must understand its technological aspects in order to utilize it better, and become acquainted with sonographic images. In order to effectively exploit the results of intraoperative ultrasonography, our experience leads us to think that close collaboration between the surgeon and the radiologist is necessary.

References

1. Eiseman B, Greenlaw RH, Gallagher JQ (1965) Localization of common duct stones by ultrasound. Arch Surg 91: 195-199
2. Hayashi S, Wagai T, Miyazawar R et al (1962) Ultrasonic diagnosis of breast tumor and cholelithiasis. West J Surg Obstet Gynecol, January-February: 34-40
3. Knight PR, Newel JA (1963) Operative use of ultrasonics in cholelithiasis. Lancet 1023-1025
4. Schlegel JU, Diggdon P, Cuellar J (1961) The use of ultrasound for localizing renal calculi. J Urol 86: 367-369

2 Physical Basis and Elementary Technology

M. Dauzat, F.-M. Lopez

2.1 Ultrasounds and Their Interactions with Tissues

2.1.1 Ultrasounds

Ultrasounds can be defined as mechanical vibrations of matter at frequencies beyond those audible to human ears (that is to say, above 20000 Hz). The frequencies most generally used in sonography range between 1000000 and 10000000 Hz (1-10 MHz).

As ultrasounds are propagated into different media, their celerity depends on the density and elastic modulus of the medium concerned. Thus, the ultrasounds' propagation celerity in biological tissues varies considerably (Fig. 2.1). It is very low in air, very high in bone, and intermediate in water. Tissues such as blood, liver, kidney, fat, etc., are penetrated by ultrasound at celerities that are close to those in water, but nonetheless slightly different in each tissue. The mean speed of ultrasound in soft tissues is 1540 m/s.

2.1.2 Interactions between Ultrasounds and Tissues

The characteristic physical differences between tissues with regard to ultrasounds (which are linked to the density and the elastic modulus) are expressed by the word *impedance* (resistance to a periodic phenomenon). When ultrasounds pass from one medium to another, they surmount an *interface* (a virtual separation limit between two media) whose qualities depend on the acoustic impedance difference between the two (in the same way as light encounters an interface when it travels from a gaseous medium, like air, to a solid medium such as glass).

At this interface, some of the ultrasound energy is transmitted (passes, in fact, through the interface), and the rest is reflected. Transmission proceeds in the initial direction if the incidence of the ultrasound wave was perpendicular to the interface (Fig. 2.2a); the reflection proceeds at the same angle (but of course in the opposite direction).

Transmission proceeds in a different direction (refraction) if the incidence was not perpendicular. The same applies to reflection (Fig. 2.2b). When the interface is formed by an object whose dimensions are small compared to the ultrasound wavelength, scattering occurs (the energy spreads out in all directions). The wave-

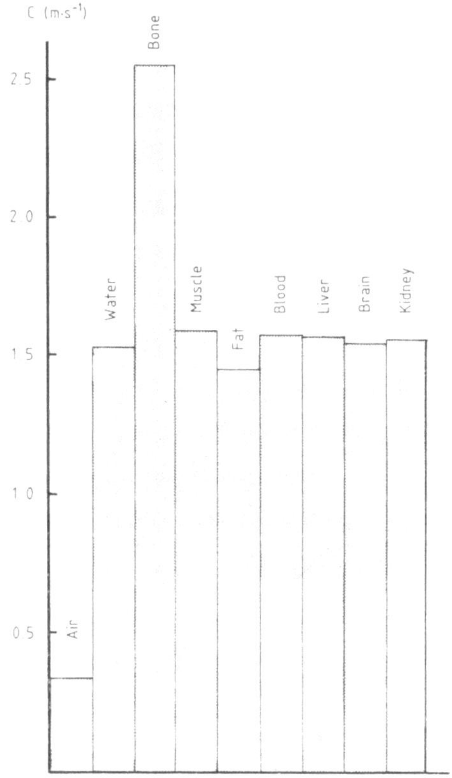

Fig. 2.1. Differences in propagation speed (celerity) of ultrasound according to the media crossed; *c* celerity ($m.s.^{-1}$)

length used in ultrasonography can be measured in millimeters. There is scattering on blood cells that is measured in micrometers (Fig. 2.2c).

The proportion of the energy that is transmitted and that which is reflected depends upon the acoustic impedance difference between the sides of the interface. Reflection is more important when the impedance difference is great.

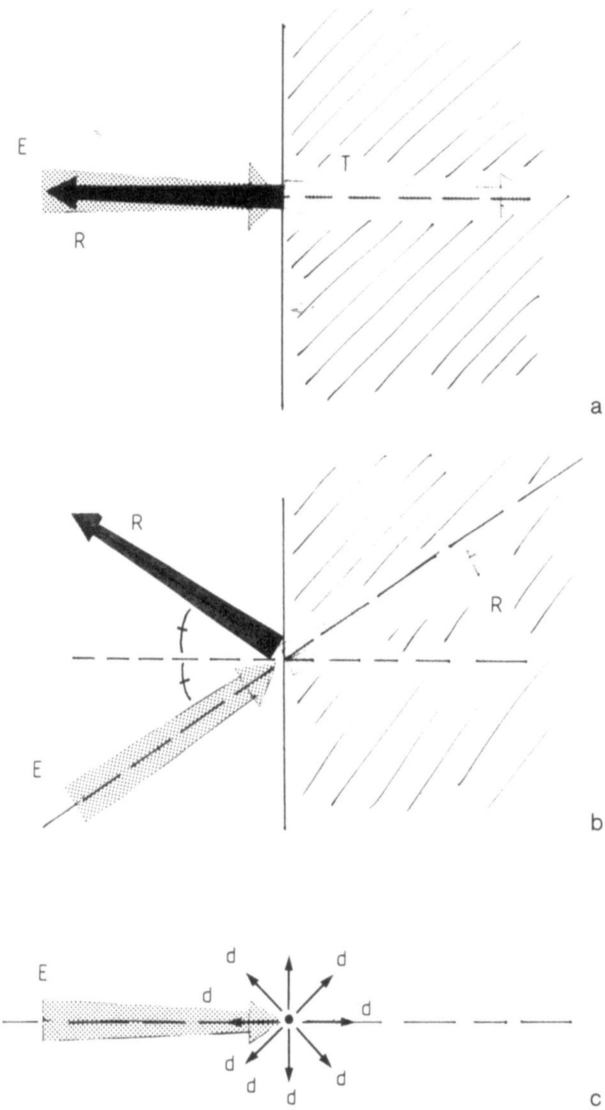

Fig. 2.2 a–c. Principal interactions of ultrasound with tissues. **a** Reflection and transmission; **b** refraction; **c** scattering. *E*, emitted energy; *R*, reflected acoustic energy; *T*, transmitted acoustic energy; *d*, scattered acoustic energy; *r*, refracted acoustic energy; *arrows* indicate direction of energy travel; *solid line*, interface; *shaded region*, second medium

2.1.3 The Ultrasound Emission and Its Echo

Morphological exploration by means of ultrasound is essentially based on reflection (echo). This means that the source of information is the acoustic energy reflected from the interfaces, which results from differences in acoustic impedance between the different adjacent tissues. The ultrasound emission is effected by a *transducer* made from a ceramic ferroelectric compound that has the ability to transduce the applied electrical energy into mechanical energy. Ultrasounds produced in this way are propagated through tissues in a preferential direction perpendicular to the transducer's surface. In B mode sonography, the emission of ultrasound is intermittent, through successive impulses separated by a time interval during which the transducer functions in reverse, that is, it transduces the reflected acoustic energy into electrical energy. Knowing the mean speed of propagation in the soft tissues (approximately 1540 m/s), it is possible to deduce the distance covered by the ultrasound impulse from the time it takes to travel it - taking into consideration the fact that the impulse must return within that time. It is, therefore, effectively an echo. Anyone can confirm this by shouting in front of a cliff; the echo occurs later, the further away the cliff is. Each interface that the ultrasound impulse meets on its way thus engenders an echo whose return delay time to the transducer is proportional to the distance separating the interface from the transducer (Fig. 2.3).

It is therefore imperative to wait for the return of the last echo (the one coming from the most distant interface) before initiating a new emission, in order to avoid an error in interpretation (confusion of a late echo from the first emission with an early echo from the second emission). In other words, the greater the distance to be explored, the longer the time interval between two emissions. The deeper the field to be explored, the more limited the number of pieces of information (sonographic images) received each second must be.

2.2 Probes and Appliances

2.2.1 Sonographic Exploration of a Spatial Dimension

If a transducer whose location is fixed emits a relatively confined ultrasound beam, the interfaces located in the path of this beam engender echoes that permit one to determine their position in that trajectory. The inflow to the transducer from each echo produces electrical information that can command the deflection of a line on an oscilloscope: we can thus obtain a unidimensional sonogram in the amplitude (A) mode (Fig. 2.4).

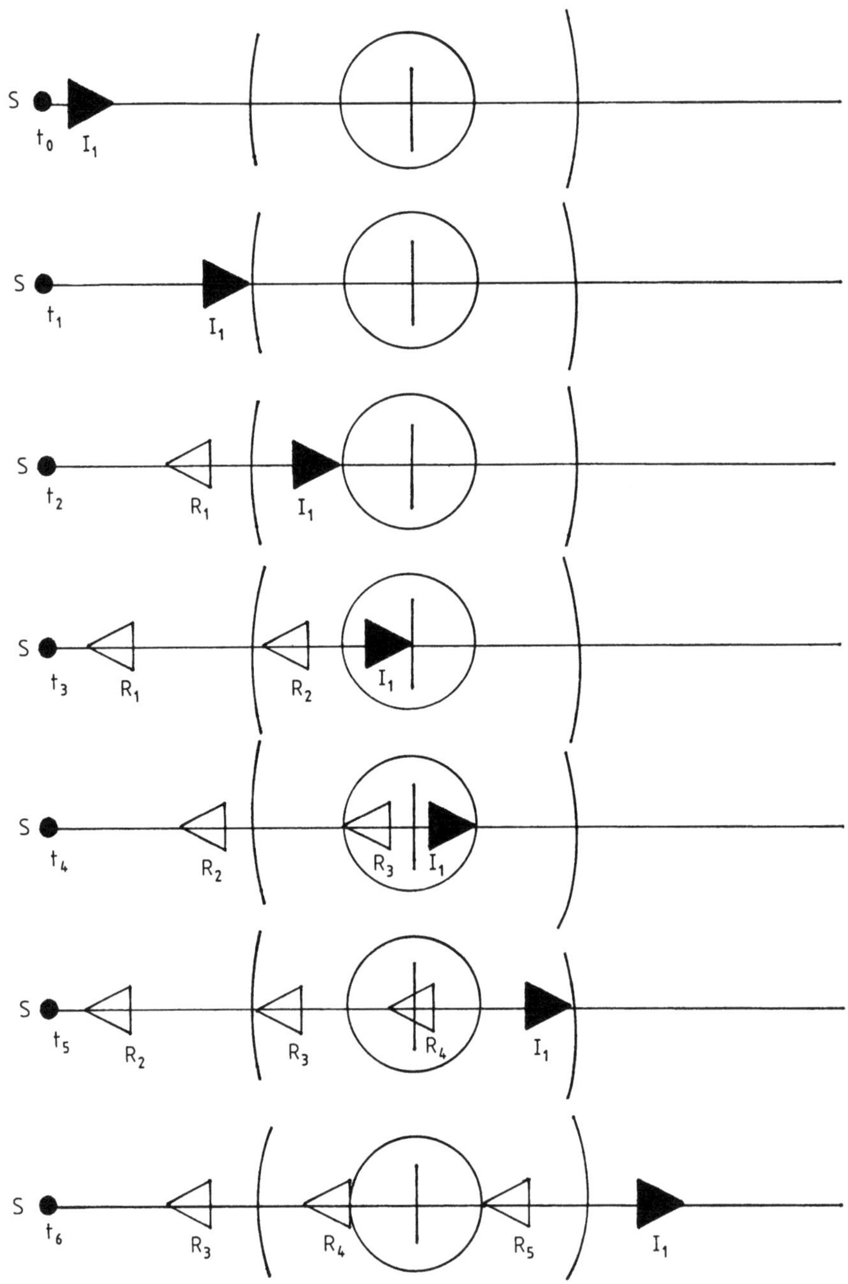

Fig. 2.3 (Legend on p. 9)

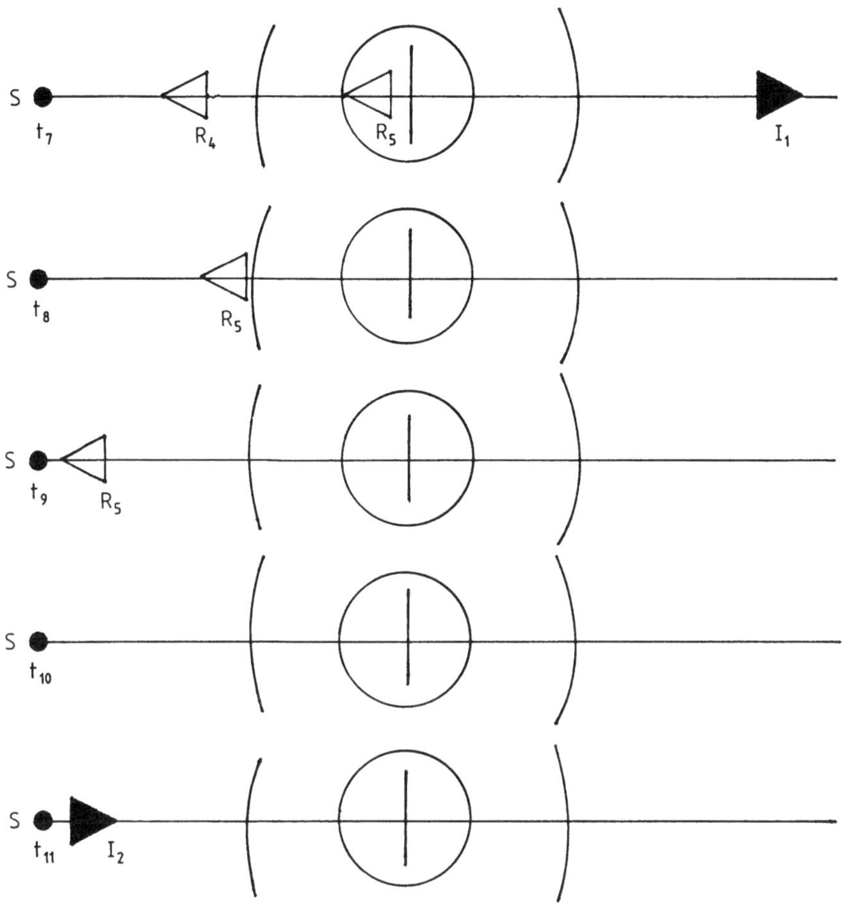

Fig. 2.3 (continued). Principles of ultrasonography. *S*, ultrasonographic probe; I_1, first acoustic pulse; t_0 to t_{11}, time; R_1 to R_5, reflected pulse (echo) of the first to fifth structures crossed; I_2, second acoustic pulse

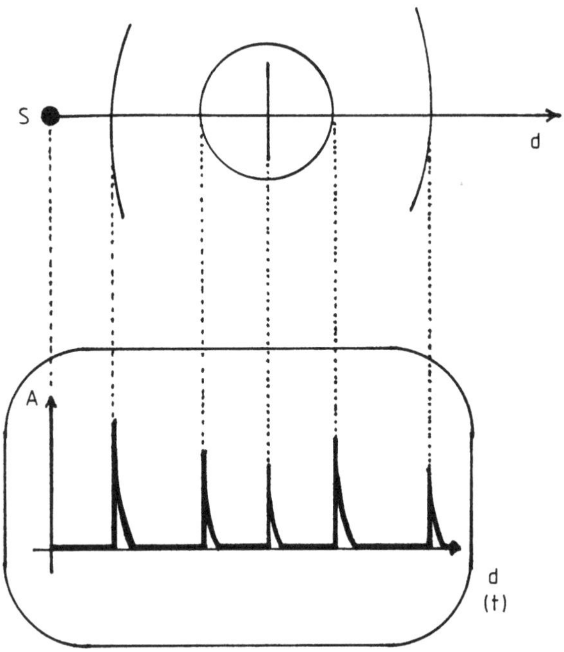

Fig. 2.4. Principles of unidimensional ultrasonography; each interface in the examined structure (*top*) generates a deflection of the horizontal line on the screen (*bottom*). *A*, amplitude of echoes; *t*, time; *d*, distance; *S*, probe

2.2.2 Significance of the Echo's Amplitude

The amplitude of the line's deflection in A-mode is related to the nature of the interface from which the echo originates. The magnitude of this amplitude depends on the difference in acoustic impedance between the sides of the interface (Fig. 2.5).

Nonetheless, when penetrating tissues, ultrasounds undergo *attenuation*, and late echoes would be weaker than early echoes, if they were not subject to greater amplification to compensate for this attenuation. This gain compensation related to the exploration depth is generally adjustable on sonographic appliances, thus enabling the differences in attenuation by the tissues being penetrated to be taken into account.

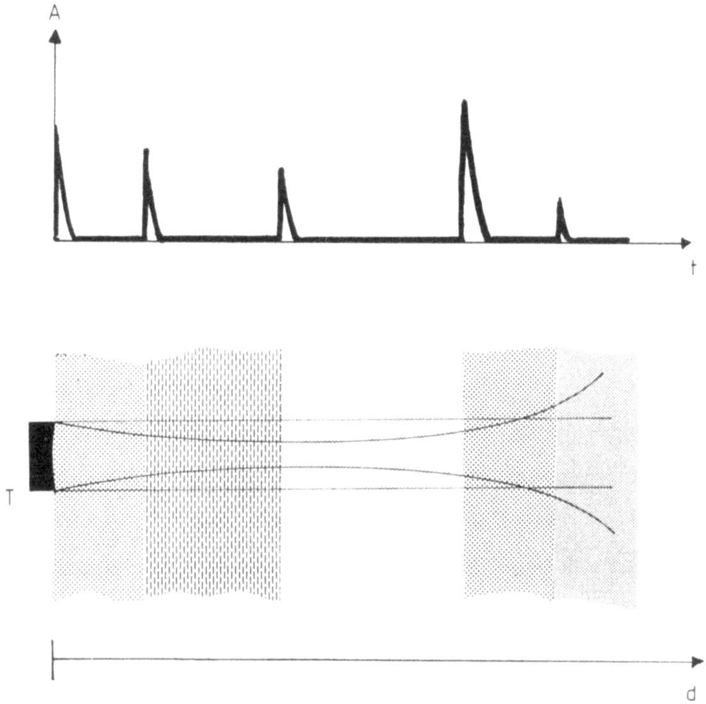

Fig. 2.5. Proportional relationship between amplitude of echoes and acoustic impedance differences constituting the reflecting interface; *T*, transducer; *A*, amplitude of echoes; *t*, time; *d*, distance

2.2.3 Brightness (B) Mode Sonography

To represent echoes on one single line, depicting the course of the ultrasound beam, it is possible to transduce the amplitude (energy) of the echo into the intensity of a luminous point placed along this line. The brightness of a point indicating the position of a structure will be dependent on the amplitude of the echo it engenders. This is the principle of brightness (B) mode sonography (Fig. 2.6).

The energy of the echo is usually represented according to a scale of gray (black for the weakest echoes, gray for echoes of intermediate energy, and white for the strongest echoes). This scale can include a variable number of levels (at least eight), and the number assigned is one of the characteristics that permit the evaluation of an sonographic appliance. Of course, a color scale can be substituted for the gray scale; as such, the substitution offers more esthetic satisfaction than it does assistance toward diagnosis; it is not used very often.

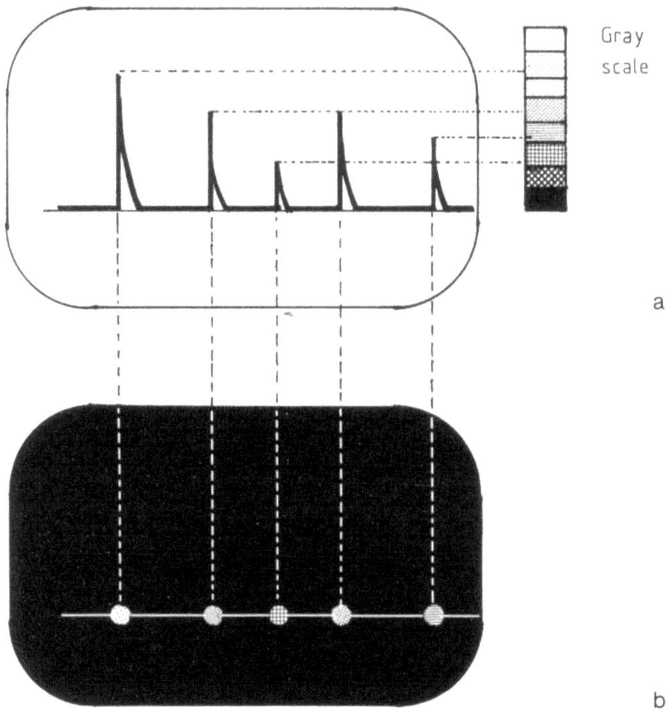

Fig. 2.6. Principles of B-(brightness) mode sonography. **a** A mode; **b** B mode. The brightness of each spot on the screen (*B mode*) is relative to the amplitude of the vertical deflection (*A mode*), i.e., to the differences in acoustic impedance constituting the interfaces

2.2.4 Bidimensional Sonography or Echotomography

If we use several ultrasound beams, or simply displace the ultrasound beams, allowing the exploration of a spatial dimension, we can, from several lines situated in the same plane, reconstitute an image in two dimensions: this is the principle of echotomography (Fig. 2.7).

2.2.5 Echotomography in B-Mode

The application of brightness (B) mode to bidimensional sonography represents the most commonly used form of echotomography (Fig. 2.8). If the number of images constructed each second is sufficient to enable the observation of mobile structural displacements (cardiac valves, for instance), we call this real-time sonography. In practice, this represents an image-realization frequency of over 12 images/s. As mentioned above, this frequency is higher when the dimensions of the field explored are restricted, and of course the more exploration lines are used, the sharper the image will be, although the reconstruction of the image will be slower if the number of lines is high.

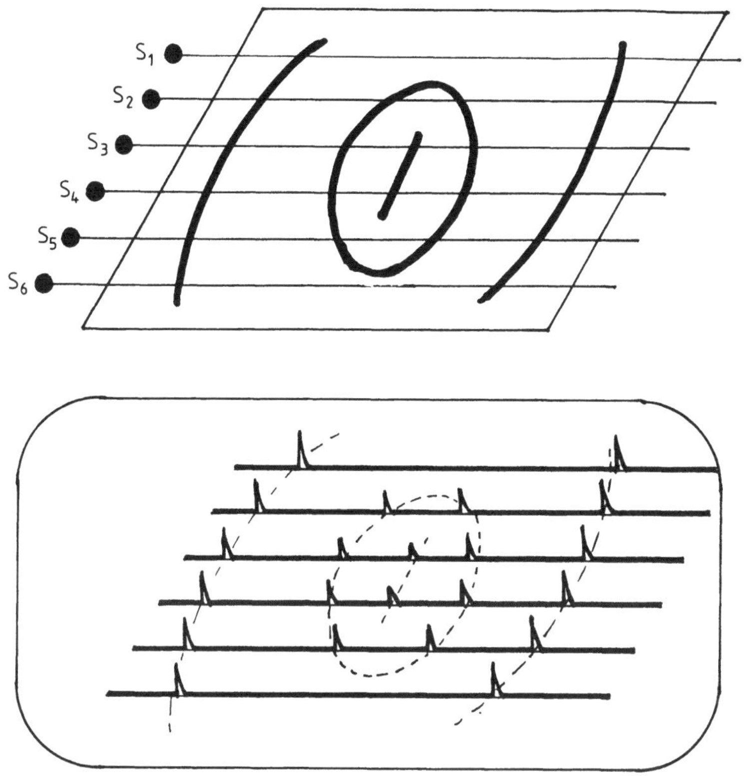

Fig. 2.7. Principles of bidimensional ultrasonography or echotomography. S_1–S_6, probes or successive positions of the probe

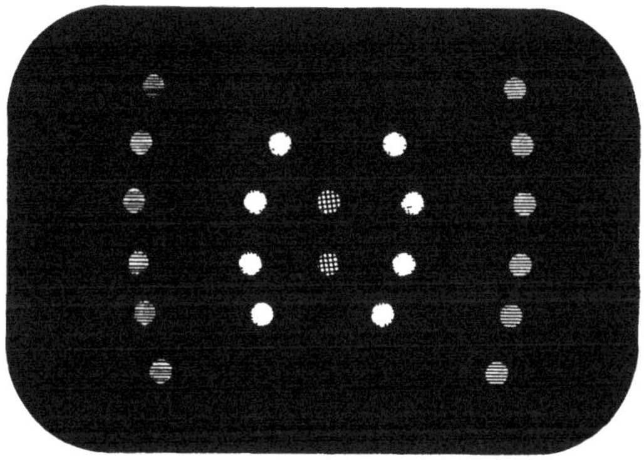

Fig. 2.8. Echotomography in B-(brightness) mode. The amplitude of echoes is coded according to a scale of luminous intensity (gray scale) ⊜, high-level echoes; ◌, intermediate-level echoes; ⊕, low-level echoes

2.2.6 Real-Time B-Mode Echotomography

Echotomography in real time will supplant totally manual static scanning from now on. Exploration in real time is the only method that is usable intraoperatively. The image constructed can be in the shape of a rectangle (linear scanning) or a sector (sector scanning; Fig. 2.9). This type of image results from the manner in which the ultrasound beam is displaced in the plane chosen for the exploration (the sweeping movement): by translation or by rotation movement about an axis.

2.2.7 Mechanical Scanning Probes

The box containing the transducer or transducers, which allows the displacement of the ultrasound beam, is called the probe. Some probes consist of a moveable transducer driven by a motor. Displacement of the ultrasound beam is then achieved by displacement of the transducer. In most cases, these probes (called mechanical scanning probes) effect echotomographic sections in sectorial form. The transducer's movement can be either rotatory (in which case several transducers can be associated) or oscillatory (Fig. 2.10).

2.2.8 Electronic Scanning Probes

Other kinds of probes are composed of many ultrasonic transducers. Displacement of the ultrasound beam is then obtained by means of an electronic commutation: the first transducer allows the build-up of a first exploration line, then passes the relay to the second, to the third, and so on. Such probes (called electronic scanning probes) do not contain any moving parts. The shape of an image constructed in this manner is usually rectangular (linear scanning); it may also be sectorial, the movement of the ultrasound beam emitted being directed by an electronic procedure (see the chapter on electronic focusing). A few convex probes perform intermediate scanning (Fig. 2.11).

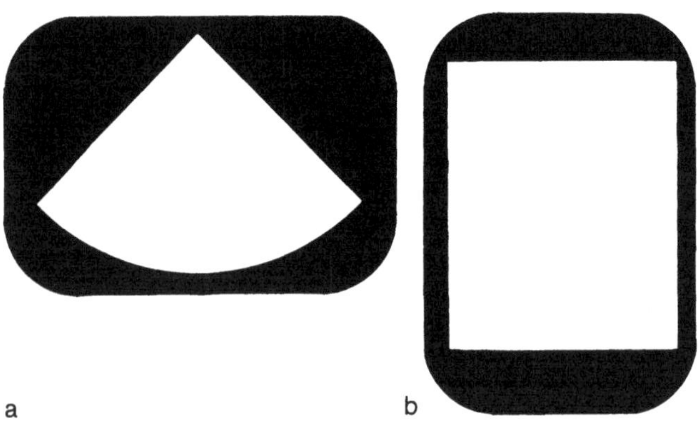

a b

Fig. 2.9 a, b. The different modes of echotomographic scanning. **a** Sectorial scanning; **b** linear scanning

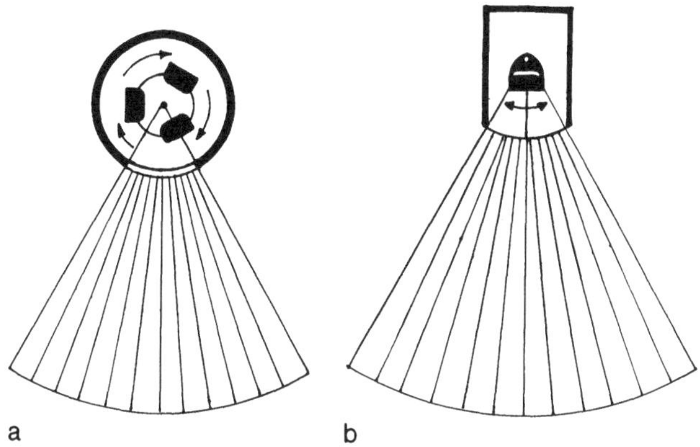

Fig. 2.10 a, b. The different types of mechanical sectorial scanning probes. **a** Rotatory probe; **b** oscillatory probe. *Arrows* indicate the motion of the transducer(s)

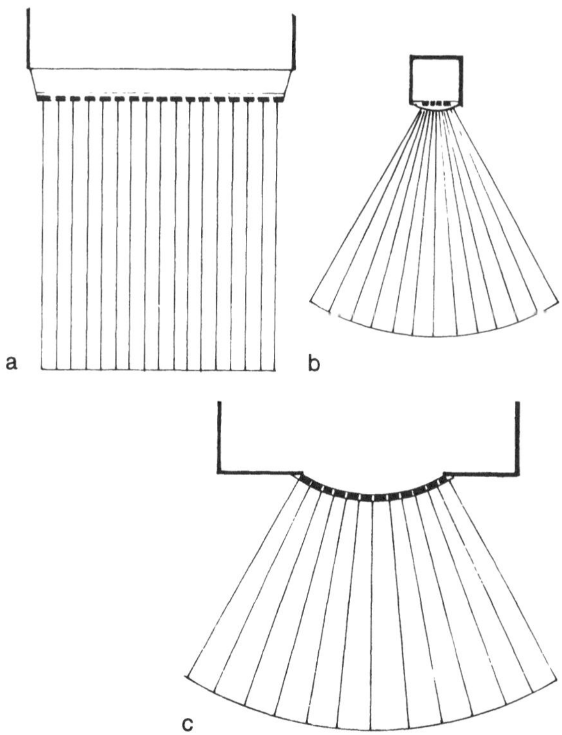

Fig. 2.11 a–c. The different types of electronic scanning probes. **a** Linear scanning; **b** Sectorial scanning; **c** Convex probe

2.2.9 The Geometry of the Ultrasound Beam

The quality of an echotomographic image depends on the resolution of the appliance: this means both contrast resolution (ability to differentiate tissues that present the smallest possible differences in acoustic impedance) and spatial resolution (ability to visualize the smallest possible structures).

The thickness of the sonographic section is one of the parameters determining the spatial resolution. It is directly linked to the geometry of the ultrasound beam transmitted by the transducer. The finer the beam, the thinner the section, and the better the echotomographic image. The ultrasound beam emitted by the transducer is not a virtual line: the acoustic energy spreads out around the axis of the beam, forming a cylinder of variable diameter (which is minimal at the focal point, and widens beyond it).

The lower the frequency of the ultrasound emission, and the smaller the transducer's diameter, the shorter will be the distance at which the beam diverges (Fig. 2.12). In other words, the most regular beams are obtained using transducers that have wide diameters and use high frequencies.

2.2.10 Acoustic Focusing

The shape of the ultrasound beam can be improved in order to obtain a thinner section: a transducer with a slightly concave surface emits a beam that is constricted at a certain distance (called the focal zone or focus), and diverges afterwards (Fig. 2.13). It is evident that the edges of an ultrasound beam are not as sharp and do not contrast as strongly as is suggested by the usual diagrammatic representation. In fact, the acoustic energy decreases progressively with increasing distance from the beam's axis (Fig. 2.13).

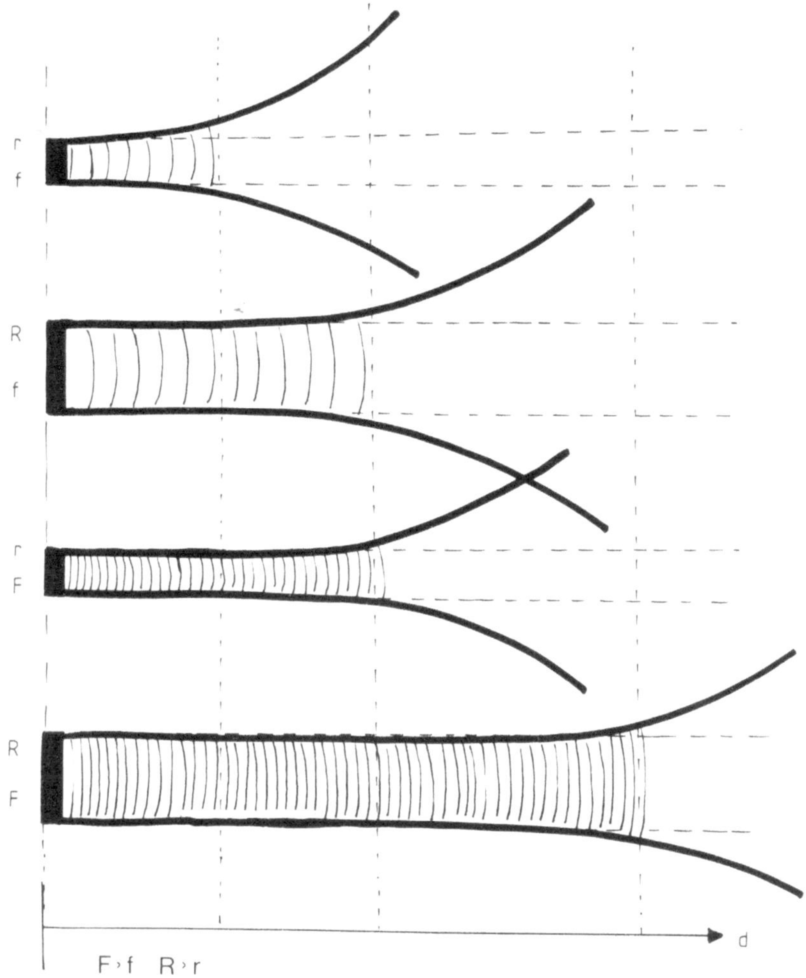

Fig. 2.12. Determination of the geometry of the ultrasound beam by the transducer's diameter and the emitting frequency; *R* and *r*, beam of the transducer ($R > r$); *F* and *f*, emitting frequency ($F > f$); *d*, distance

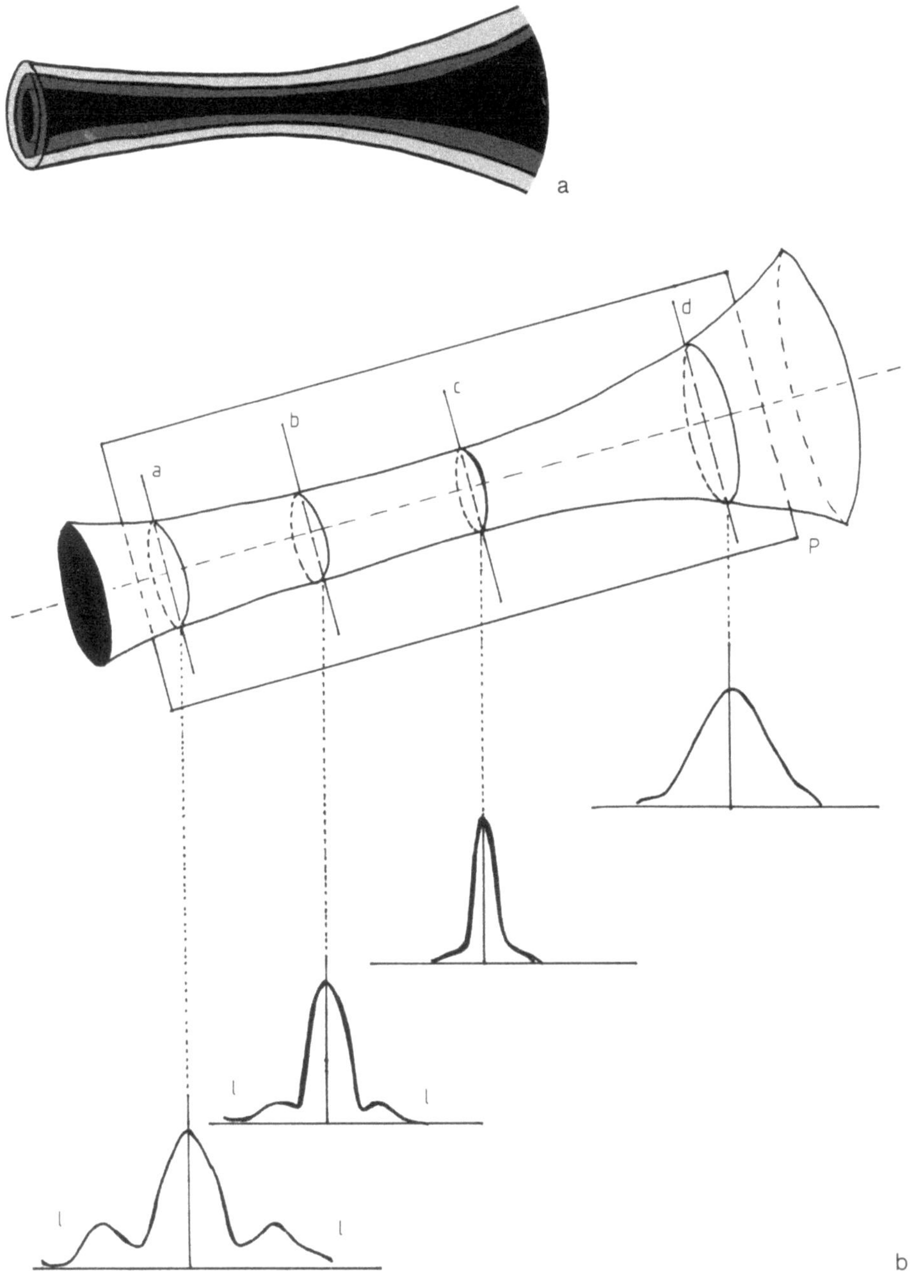

Fig. 2.13 a, b. Modification of the form of the ultrasound beam by acoustic focusing. **a** The distribution of the acoustic energy decreases when we move away from the beam's axis (here represented by decreasing gray intensities). **b** Tridimensional representation of the beam showing the variations in distribution of the acoustic energy (*top*), and energy amplitude on both sides of the beam axis (*lines a–d in the P plane*). Notice, in the *proximal zone*, the presence of "lateral lobes" (*l*), which can cause artifacts on the sonographic images when they come across very echogenic structures

2.2.11 Focusing and Resolution

As a consequence, the geometry of the ultrasound beam determines the spatial resolution in directions that are perpendicular to the axis of the ultrasound beam. When building up an exploration line to form an echotomographic image, structures situated along the axis of the ultrasound beam will be represented by points, whose luminous intensities are linked to the quality of the interface, but whose dimensions are constant, whereas those of the ultrasound beam are not (Fig. 2.14). Reflective targets of different dimensions can thus be represented in the same way (Fig. 2.14a, b). On the other hand, targets relatively distant from the beam's axis can be falsely interpreted as being located in the axis if they are not located within the area of best focus (Fig. 2.14c).

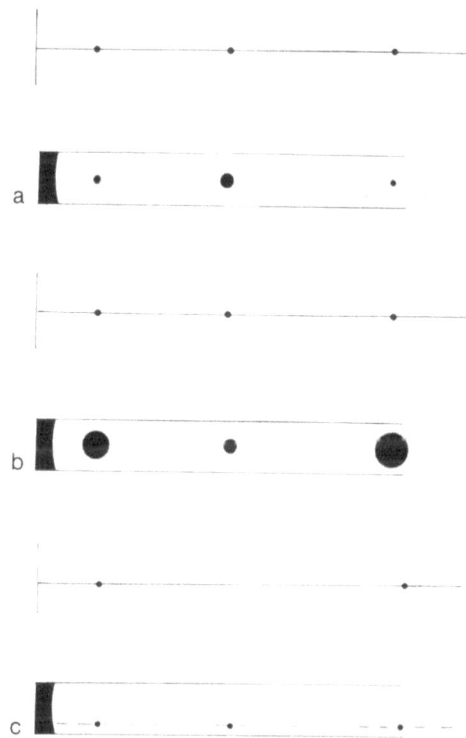

Fig. 2.14a–c. Focusing and lateral resolution. **a, b** Structures of different dimensions can be represented in the same way if they are included in the lateral limits of the beam. **c** Structures located far away from the beam's axis are not taken into account in the focal zone, but can be taken into account in the proximal and distal zones where the beam is divergent. In **a–c**, (*bottom*) echogenic structures (*dots*) of different size and position with respect to the ultrasound beam (*shaded areas*); (*top*) B-mode representation of echoes generated by these structures

2.2.12 Duration of the Ultrasound Pulse Emitted

Acoustic damping and sensitivity characteristics depend upon the quality of the transducer and its associated materials (particularly the supporting structures). A sensitive transducer is able to detect echoes of low intensity. A well-damped transducer is capable of transmitting very short ultrasound pulses. This shortness is essential for good axial spatial resolution. Besides the backing materials associated with the transducer, the emission frequency (itself dependent on the transducer's thickness) determines the duration of the pulse. The shortest pulses are obtained with the highest emission frequencies (Fig. 2.15). Consequently, the best sonograms will be provided by high-frequency probes. Unfortunately, high-frequency ultrasound is subjected to much more significant attenuation in the tissues than low-frequency ultrasound is. Therefore, the use of these high-frequency probes is only practically possible for exploration of superficial organs.

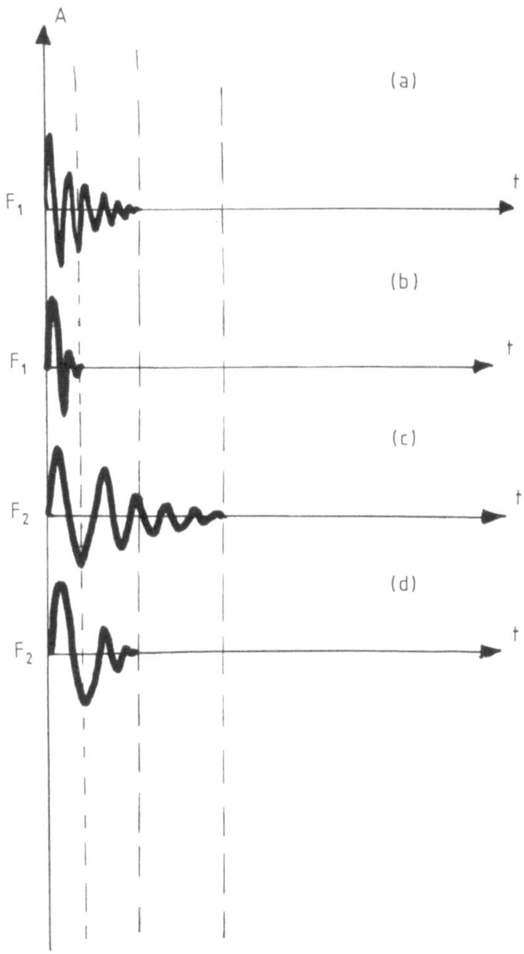

Fig. 2.15. Association between duration of the ultrasound pulse transmitted, the frequency of the emission, and the qualities of the material associated with the transducer (damping). *A*, amplitude; *t*, time; F_1, high frequency; F_2, low frequency; *a*, high frequency with poor damping; *b*, high frequency with good damping; *c*, low frequency with bad damping; *d*, low frequency with good damping

2.2.13 Volume of the Ultrasound Pulse

The acoustic energy sent out by the transducer is concentrated in the ultrasound beam, whose axis is perpendicular to the transducer's surface. As mentioned above, this beam is not perfectly cylindrical but diverges in its distal portion and can be constricted in the focal zone if the transducer's surface is so disposed as to determine focusing. The discharged ultrasound pulse is propagated along the beam's axis, following its variations in diameter. The acoustic energy is accumulated in a volume that is the shape of a pear whose length (axial dimension) is constant during its course but whose width (lateral dimensions) changes according to the focus (Fig. 2.16).

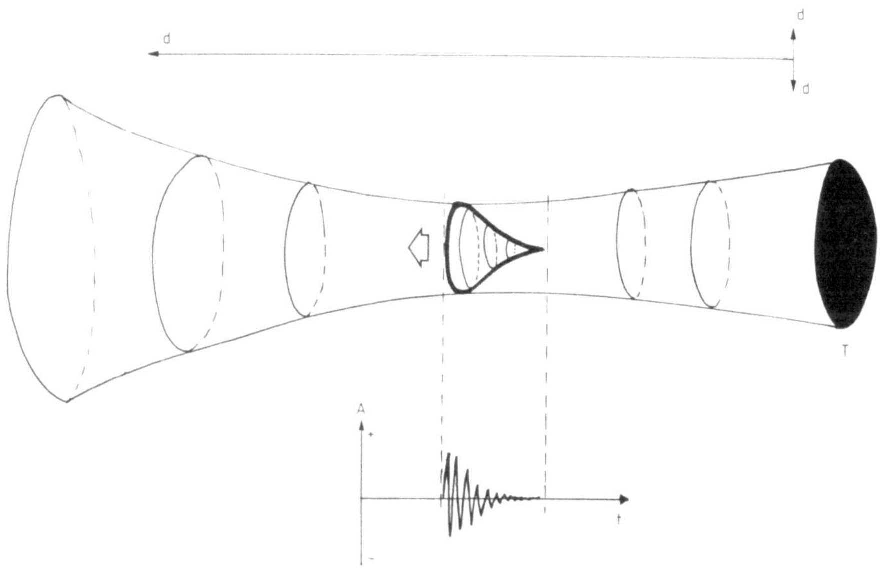

Fig. 2.16. Shape and dimensions of the ultrasound impulse. The pulse has the shape of a pear whose lateral dimensions vary along the course of the beam, whereas its axial dimension remains constant. (*Top*) tridimensional representation of the pulse and beam. (*Bottom*) amplitude-time diagram of pulse (see Fig. 2.15). *T*, transducer; *d*, distance; *A*, amplitude; *large arrow*, direction of propagation; (+), positive; (−), negative

2.2.14 Duration of the Pulse and Axial Resolution

The axial resolution corresponds to the smallest distance between two close structures in the same direction as the ultrasound beams used, that the sonograph remains able to differentiate. The duration of the pulse directly affects this resolution: if the pulse is long, the axial resolution is weak (Fig. 2.17). We have noted that the higher the transmission frequency and the better the transducer is damped, the shorter the pulse can be. In other words, a high-frequency transducer that is badly damped does not permit as good an axial spatial resolution as a transducer of lower frequency but with a good damping coefficient. The frequency represents, therefore, an important element in the choice of a probe; however, it is not the only determinant of its quality.

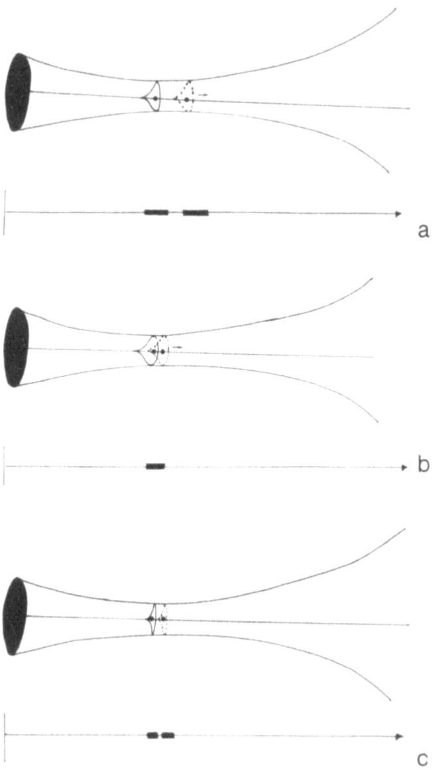

Fig. 2.17 a–c. Effect of impulse duration on axial resolution. **a** Two close structures (*dots*) can be distinguished if the distance separating them is greater than the axial dimension of the pulse. **b** They are not distinguished from each other if this distance is less. **c** A shorter pulse allows them to be distinguished. (*Top*) representation of ultrasound beam and pulses; (*bottom*) B-mode representation of the resulting echoes; *arrow*, direction of propagation

2.2.15 Axial Resolution is Constant Along the Beam

As described in Sect. 2.2.11, the resolution perpendicular to the axis of the ultrasound beam varies with the geometry of the beam, being optimal in the focal area (Fig. 2.14). In contrast, the axial resolution, which directly depends on the duration of the ultrasound pulse, is constant along the beam (Fig. 2.18) because the duration does not vary.

2.2.16 Electronic Scanning Focusing

The lateral dimensions of the ultrasound beam thus depend on the transmission frequency, the diameter of the beam, and the form of the transducer. Electronic scanning probes can improve lateral resolution within the plane of section via electronic focusing achieved by functionally linking several transducers. The construction of an exploration line is then no longer performed by only one transduc-

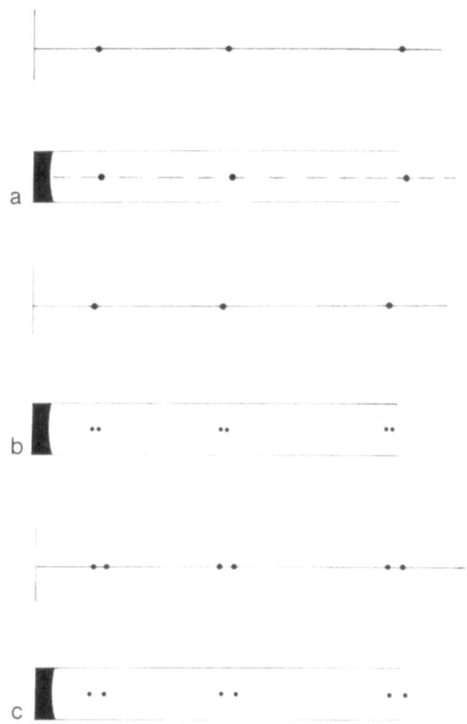

Fig. 2.18 a–c. The axial resolution is constant along the beam. **a** Identical structures engender identical images along this axis. **b** Structures that are too close are not distinguished. **c** Less close to each other, structures can be distinguished whatever their position on the beam's course may be

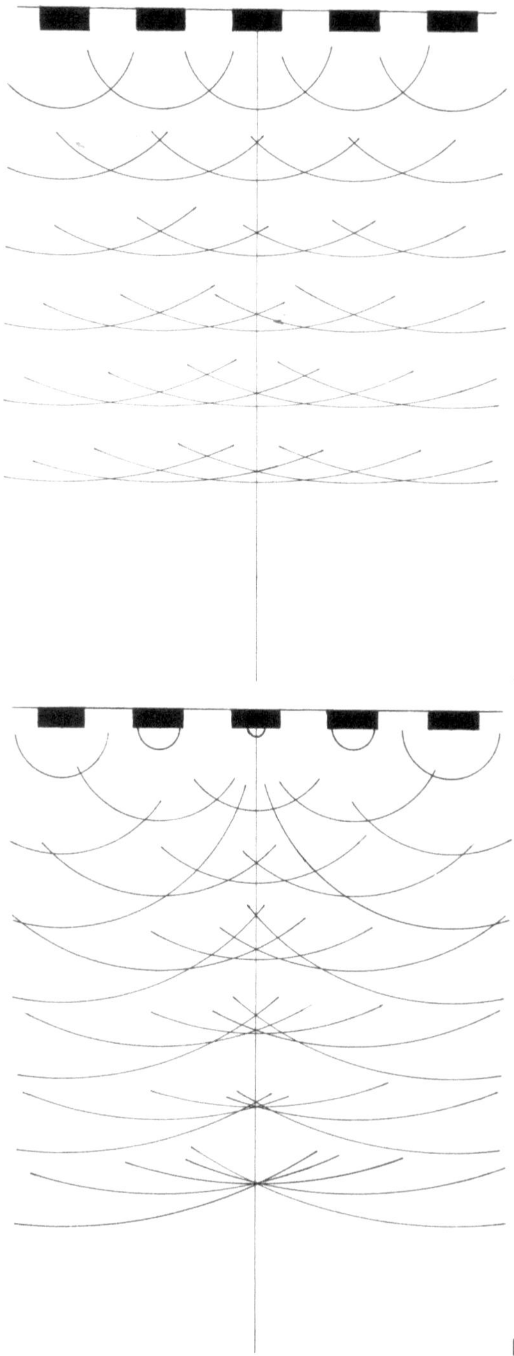

a

b

Fig. 2.19 a, b. Principles of electronic focusing. A group of transducers (in this case five) is required for the construction of an exploration line. **a** If the emission is simultaneous, the wave front is a plane parallel to the surface of the probe. **b** If the emission is out of phase, the acoustic energy can be synchronized (concentrated) at one point

er, but by a group of transducers. If all the transducers emit simultaneously, the acoustic energy is distributed as a wave front parallel to the probe's surface. However, if the emission of each transducer is slightly out of phase, it is possible to obtain, at specific moments in time, a nonuniform distribution of acoustic energy. If the intervals between emissions are well adjusted, the acoustic energy can be concentrated at one point (Fig. 2.19). What is possible at the point of emission is also possible at the point of reception, so that echoes coming from targets located at this electronic focusing point are relatively increased in intensity and amplification. In the extreme, an exploration line can be built up from several points (or, more precisely, several zones, because the focusing is not really to a point) by transmitting successive differently focused pulses along this line: "pursuit focusing", which provides excellent images. In terms of lateral resolution, this requires the expenditure of a long image-construction time, as well as heavier and more expensive electronic appliances.

The same procedure that enables the concentration of acoustic energy within one zone, by manipulating emission intervals within a group of transducers, can be utilized for "ultrasound-beam deviation" and thus allow different types of scanning. In this manner, a linear, sectorial, or even trapezoidal scan can be obtained from an electronic probe (Fig. 2.11). The technique of electronic focusing can also be applied to mechanical scanning probes; in this case the transducer is sectioned into concentric rings (annular-array-focused probes). Such probes are not yet popular, but are rapidly becoming accepted. In comparison with simple acoustic focusing obtained by adapting the transducer's surface (concavity), electronic focusing has the advantage of being adjustable. Moreover, on some probes, acoustic and electronic focusing are combined.

2.2.17 Spatial Resolution and Scanning Mode

Spatial resolution is thus assessed according to three dimensions: axial resolution (A) in the axis of the beam, lateral resolution (L) perpendicular to this axis within the plane of section, and resolution in thickness perpendicular to the axis of the beam and to the plane of section (E). The axial resolution is constant within the field explored, which is rectangular as well as sectorial (except for the proximal zone immediately underneath the probe, from which information can generally not be well extracted). The lateral resolution is poor outside these zones.

In mechanical sectorial scanning systems, lateral resolution is limited by the number of lines per unit of surface. With this sectorial scanning, the density of the lines per surface unit is more important in the proximal area; at increasing distances from the probe, the lateral resolution becomes less accurate. Resolution of thickness is mainly dependent upon the type of ultrasound beam used, as it results from acoustic focusing. It is therefore optimal in the focal zone and deteriorates on either side (Fig. 2.20).

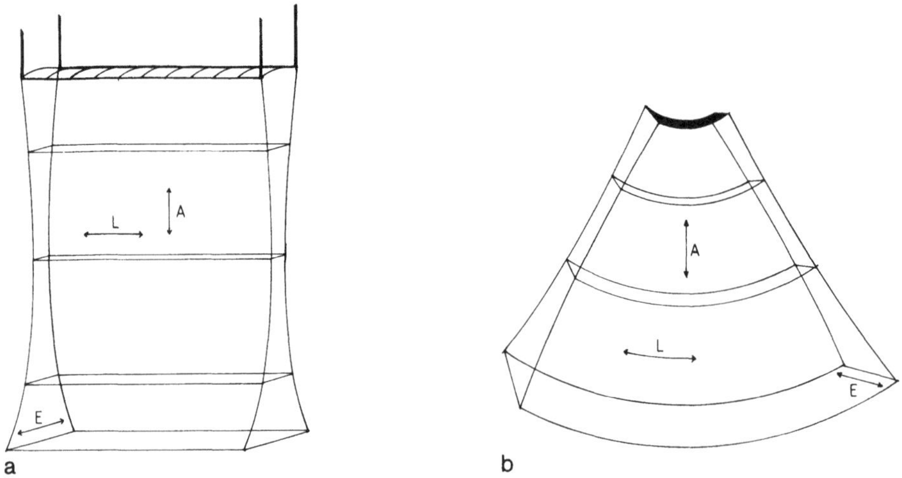

Fig. 2.20 a, b. Spatial resolution in linear **a** and sectorial **b** scanning. *A*, axial resolution; *L*, lateral resolution; *E*, resolution in thickness

2.3 Practical Bases for Utilization

2.3.1 Representation of Sonograms

The conventions for representation of sonographic images are the following:

1. The echoes are shown in white on a black background (the more echogenic the structure is, i.e., the greater the differences in acoustic impedance between the sides of the interface, the more brilliant the image obtained on the screen is).
2. The front (anterior or ventral surface) of the patient is represented at the top of the screen.
3. The back (posterior or dorsal surface) is represented in the lower part of the screen.
4. The right side of the patient is shown on the left of the screen, and the left side of the patient is shown on the right. Consequently, a transverse horizontal section is represented as if it were seen from below (using the same convention that applies to X-ray scans).
5. The patient's head (the top, or cephalic pole) is depicted on the left of the screen, and the feet (lower part, or caudal pole) on the right of the screen: a sagittal longitudinal section is similarly represented (with the head of the patient on the left) if the patient is in the supine or the prone position. Conforming to this convention is important, in order to facilitate the interpretation of sonograms (Fig. 2.21).

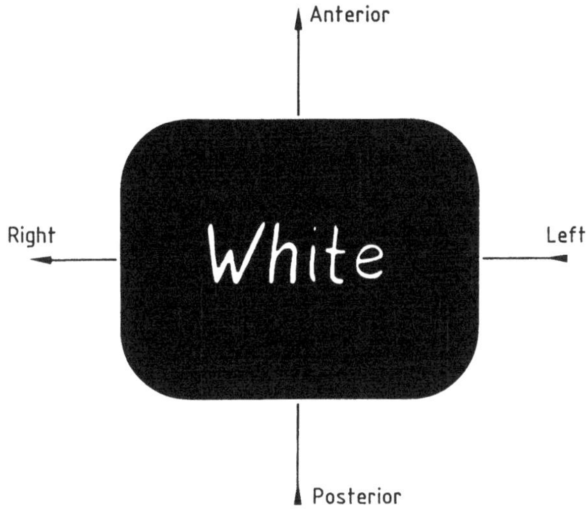

Fig. 2.21. Convention for representation of sonographic images

2.3.2 Basic Sonographic Signs (Glossary)

So, acoustic energy is transformed into luminous intensity on the sonographic screen. Strong acoustic energies are represented by high intensities, and the weak energies by the low intensities (black). The acoustic energy of the echo is termed *echogenicity*. Such a notion is a relative one. The echogenicity of a structure is compared with that of adjacent structures, and described as follows:

1. Isoechogenic structures are of the same echogenicity as their environment.
2. Hyperechogenic structures are more echogenic than their environment.
3. When hyperechogenic structures stop the ultrasound beam (strong absorption), no structure can be visualized deep to them anymore: they produce an *acoustic shadow*. This is the case, for instance, with osseous structures, which practically cannot be penetrated by ultrasounds. The acoustic shadow of the ribs is a classic obstacle to the examination of the thoracic portion of the liver.
4. Hypoechogenic structures are less echogenic than their environment.
5. Anechogenic structures give no visible echo.
6. If a structure is very anechogenic, it produces less significant ultrasound attenuation than occurs within the surrounding structures, so that the beam traversing this anechogenic structure engenders afterwards more intensive echoes than the beam that has passed through the adjacent structures. This is referred to as *posterior reinforcement* or *facilitation*. Occurrence of this phenomenon is consistent with the liquid nature of an anechogenic structure (Fig. 2.22).

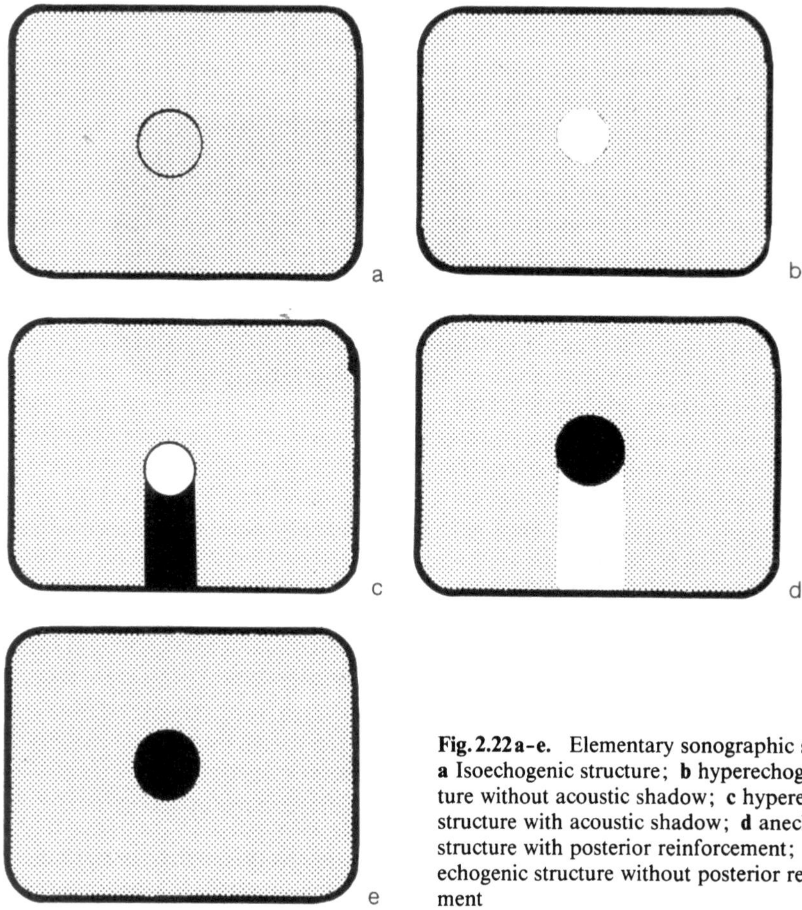

Fig. 2.22 a–e. Elementary sonographic signs. **a** Isoechogenic structure; **b** hyperechogenic structure without acoustic shadow; **c** hyperechogenic structure with acoustic shadow; **d** anechogenic structure with posterior reinforcement; **e** anechogenic structure without posterior reinforcement

2.3.3 Pitfalls and Artifacts in the Construction of a Sonogram

Certain features of the construction of a sonographic image are important:

1. An acoustic shadow can partially or totally obscure an underlying structure (Fig. 2.23 a).
2. The lateral parts of a rounded structure are usually not visualized clearly. This is due to the so-called *tangency* phenomenon, which, as a result of diffraction, deflects the ultrasound beam when the reflected component is very weak (Fig. 2.23 b).
3. The refraction that appears when the ultrasound beam traverses a relatively thick structure with an acoustic impedance that is considerably different from that of the surrounding structures can deflect the ultrasound beam so that a distally situated structure will be represented in an erroneous position. This artifact occurs only when the ultrasound beam strikes the structure responsible for refraction at an oblique angle of incidence (Fig. 2.23 c). The latter phenomenon

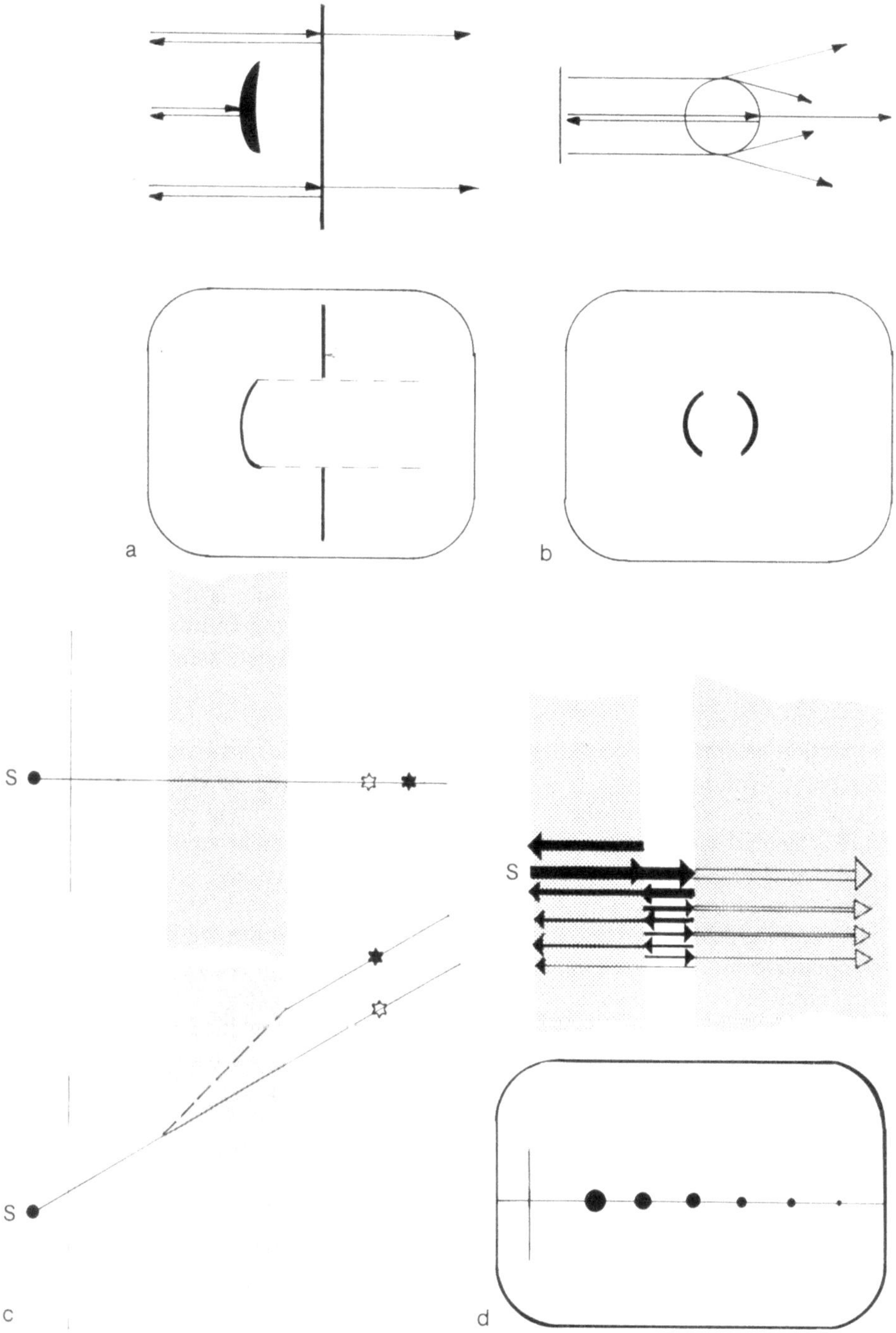

Fig. 2.23 a–d. The main sonographic artifacts. **a–d** (*Top*) echogenic structures and ultrasound direction of propagation (*arrows*); (*bottom*) B-mode sonogram. **a** Acoustic shadow; **b** the phenomenon of tangency; *S*, source; **c** refraction (if full, the real position of the structure, if empty, the position marked on the screen). At the *top*, the error of distance evaluation without deviation of the beam, which can result from the differences in propagation speed of the ultrasound according to the structures crossed. **d** Repetition echo

can hamper the guidance of a puncture, if only external markers are used. Its effects can be corrected by maintaining visualization of the needle and the structure to be punctured with the same probe.

4. Two parallel interfaces that are successively traversed by the ultrasound beam can trap the acoustic pulse, which will undergo multiple reflections between them. A single structure may create several different echoes that appear to be regularly spaced while their intensity decreases at a regular rate. This classical artifact is called *repetition echo,* and is easily detectable by its characteristic "scale" appearance. It may be found deep to an anechogenic structure, e.g., a cyst (Fig. 2.23 d).

2.3.4 Different Probes for Intraoperative Use

It is impossible to list all the different probes available for intraoperative use, as progress in this field has been rapid and significant. The most recent probes are of the linear electronic scanning type. The classical example is the "slide" probe (Fig. 2.24 a), which is, however, more suitable for percutaneous exploration. Less cumbersome models (Fig. 2.24 b, c) that resemble a hand-held safety razor are better adapted. The active face is perpendicular to the cable axis, which permits exploration of zones that are difficult to approach. Depending on the case, the plane of section may be situated in the same plane as the cable axis or in a perpendicular plane. The latter type (Fig. 2.24 b) is perfectly suited to exploration of the diaphragmatic surface of the liver. With other linear scanning probes, the active face is aligned with the connective cable. These probes can be equipped with a device that closely fits the sonographer's finger, allowing virtual "ultrasound palpation" even of the regions that are very difficult to approach, such as peritoneal recesses (Fig. 2.24 d). Finally, some sectorial scanning probes are designed for intraoperative use; they are generally supplied with a removable or fixed "water bag", enabling the transducer to be kept distant from the face of the probe, which is in direct contact with the organ to be examined. This method yields sharp images from the surface inward, and the scanning, in spite of being sectorial, presents very little divergence. This type of probe is not as easy to handle, and is principally used in vascular surgery (Fig. 2.24 e).

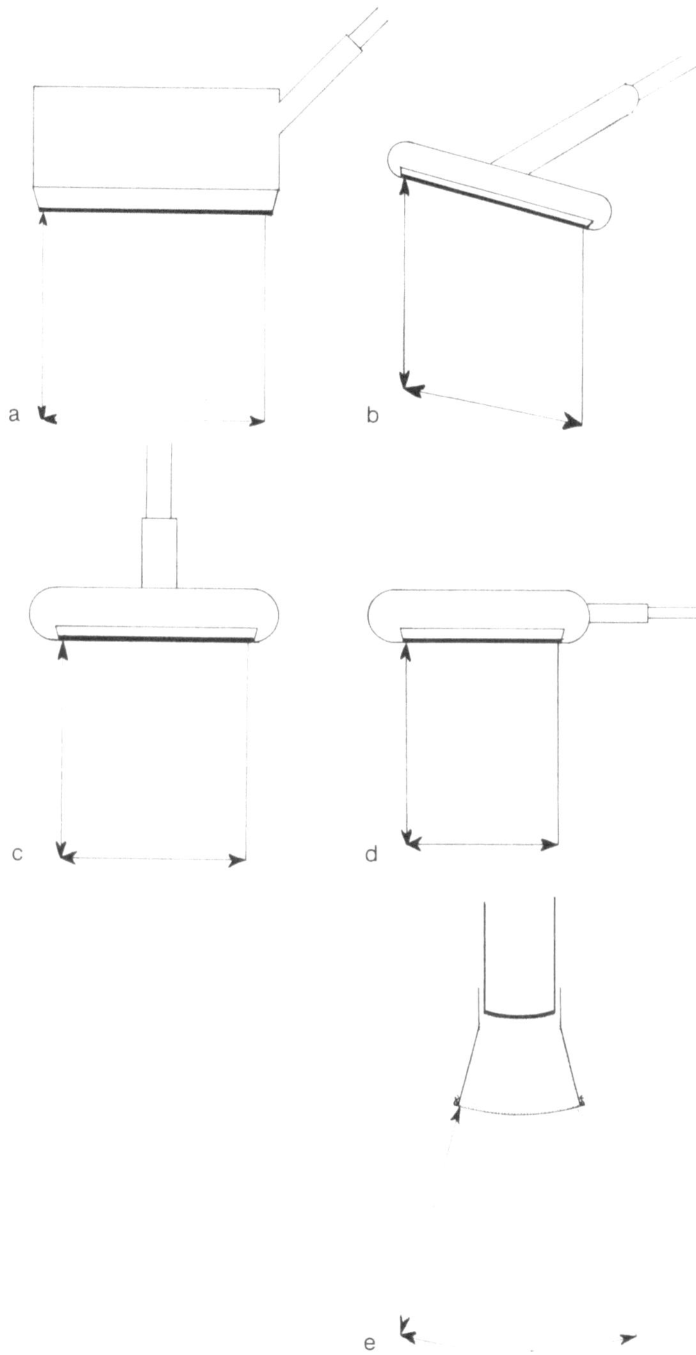

Fig. 2.24 a–e. The different probes for intraoperative use. **a** "Slide" type; **b, c** "razor" type; **d** "finger" type; **e** sectorial probe with water bag

2.3.5 Recommendations for the Manipulation of Sonographic Equipment

The routine adjustments of an echotomographic appliance intended for intraoperative use are necessarily not very numerous. Adjustment of the video screen for visualization of echotomographic images in relation to the illumination of the room should be carried out prior to the procedure, and should not be modified afterward. The presence of a scale representing the different gray levels available (from black to white), on one of the image sides, makes this adjustment much easier: it suffices to adjust the luminosity and contrast so that all the levels of this gray scale are perfectly visible and easily discernible from each other.

The gain is usually adjusted by employing a general gain button; the gain can then be adjusted in order to compensate for the ultrasound attenuation, by employing several potentiometers, each of which determine the gain for a given depth (time gain compensation, TGC). The easiest method is to place the probe on the organ to be examined and to adjust the gain to the maximum depth that is to be visualized, then to reduce the general gain to the minimum level at which this visualization is maintained, and finally to adjust the gain to an intermediate depth in order to keep the mean luminous intensity of the image almost constant at different depths (for identical anatomic structures). For instance, the proximal gain should be reduced to traverse a liquid-containing structure like the bladder.

If adjustment of the dynamic amplification can be achieved, its use is more empirical. In general, it is convenient to fix the adjustment at the position which allows slight differences in echogenicity between two structures to be distinguished. For instance, such an adjustment is useful for the detection of a hepatic metastasis which could be masked by a different adjustment (with more "contrast"). The aim is to obtain an image that is rich in information rather than a "beautiful image."

2.3.6 Equipment for Sonographically Guided Punctures

In our practice, we use three types of needle for sonographically guided peroperative punctures (Fig. 2.25). The familiar needle made by Chiba allows the puncture-injection of cystic and ductal cavities and cell-sampling by aspiration. It is atraumatic because of its very thin (22-gauge) caliber, and can be used, without running any risks, in pancreatic surgery.

Menghini-type biopsy needles can be used for the same purposes. However, they are easier to manipulate for cytodiagnosis, because of their unique fitting on a watertight syringe. They are 15- to 23-gauge in caliber, and 100–230 mm long. They can therefore be used for the liver and the pancreas.

Tru-cut needles are no longer used as frequently as the preceding types for taking samples for cytology, but are used for tissue biopsy. Because they produce more trauma, they are preferably only used for hepatic mass punctures.

The technique of sonographically guided puncture is simple in principle. In practice, the difficulty lies in simultaneously visualizing the mass or cavity to be punctured and the needle on the screen. The needle must remain within the ultrasound beam, where it appears as a series of brilliant hyperechogenic points. In order to maintain the needle in the ultrasound beam and, consequently, its image on the screen, some manufacturers have equipped their probes with guides. The guide may be a simple orifice in the slide itself (Fig. 2.26) or fixed as an accessory on the slide. The latter system usually permits frontal and lateral punctures at different angles (Fig. 2.27), and manipulations are therefore easier.

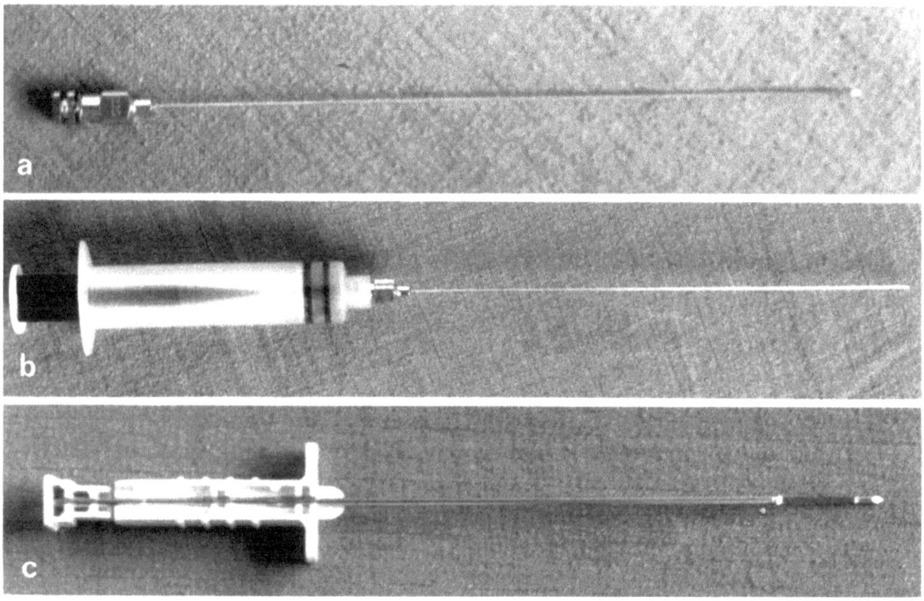

Fig. 2.25 a–c. Needle for puncture. **a** Needle from Chiba; **b** Menghini needle; **c** Tru-cut needle

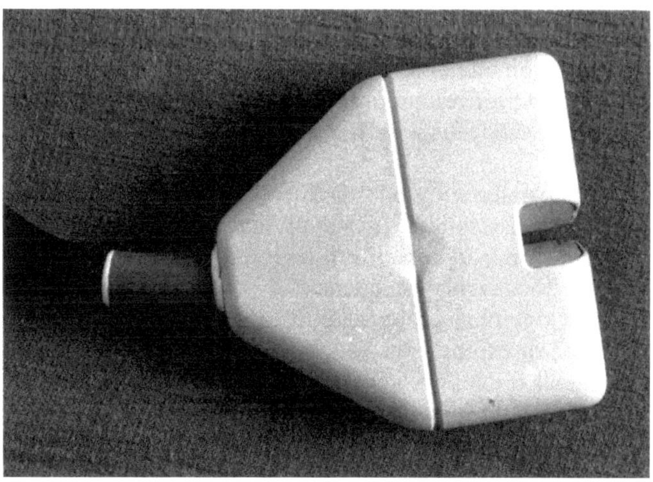

Fig. 2.26. Probe equipped with central orifice for passage of puncture needle

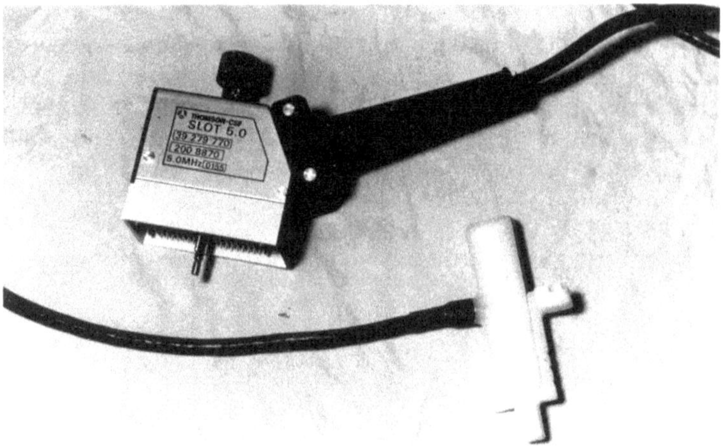

Fig. 2.27. Probe with removable needle-case guide

2.3.7 Points to Remember in Practice

- The sonogram is based on the differences in acoustic impedance between tissues; the greater these differences are, the more the resulting interfaces are enhanced.
- Bidimensional sonography provides images of anatomic sections. The luminous intensity of the points forming the image is proportional to the echogenicity of the structures reflecting the ultrasounds.
- The shape of the section is (essentially) rectangular or sectorial according to the scanning module of the probe.
- Scanning (movement of an ultrasound beam) may be achieved by mechanical or electronic means.
- The quality of the sonogram depends on the contrast resolution and the spatial resolution attained.
- The contrast resolution permits the discrimination of structures that have very similar echogenicities. It is expressed by a variable number of levels on the gray scale.
- The spatial resolution is defined in three spatial dimensions.
- The axial resolution is mainly dependent on the emission frequency. The best resolution is obtained with high frequencies.
- Nonetheless, high frequencies do not reach the deepest structures; the choice of a sonographic probe requires a compromise between the resolution and the depth of exploration.
- Lateral resolution, and resolution in thickness, depend on the geometry of the ultrasound beam. They can be improved by focusing.
- Focusing is achieved by adjustment of the transducer's surface, ("acoustic focusing") and/or by electronic control of a group of several transducers working together ("electronic focusing").

- The representation of sonograms is defined by convention.
- The terms used in sonography are based on the concept of echogenicity, e.g., hyper-, iso-, hypo-, anechogenicity, hyperechogenicity with or without acoustic shadow, and hypoechogenicity with or without reinforcement. We are also interested in the homogeneity of the structures visualized (echostructure).
- Some artifacts can detract from the sonogram, e.g., acoustic shadow phenomena, refraction, tangency, repetition echo, etc.
- The surgeon has to choose his intraoperative sonographic probe from within a very wide range. His criteria are the resolution (and consequently the frequency) but also the shape and dimensions of the field to be explored and the ergonomic convenience of the probe.

3 Ultrasonography of the Liver

B. Deixonne, M. Makuuchi, J. Mouroux, A. Pissas

3.1 Introduction

Until recent years, the surgeon who was interested in hepatic surgery had, as tools for intraoperative exploration of the liver, only his own eyes, his hands, or opacification of the biliary ducts (cholangiography) or vascular structures (ileoportography). His eyes allowed discovery of superficial lesions, his hands gave clues as to deeper ones. Biliary or vascular opacification enabled detection of lesions close to those structures that were either invading or compressing them, but certain small lesions may have evaded careful, well-managed attempts to detect them. The rise of intraoperative ultrasonography has presented the surgeon with a powerful additional weapon. Sonographic examination has proved to be as important for the clinical diagnosis of parenchymatous lesions as it is for the therapy of such lesions.

At the diagnostic stage, intraoperative sonography can permit discovery of benign or malignant lesions that may sometimes be completely overlooked during preoperative examination. At the therapeutic stage, it can direct the treatment of primary or secondary neoplastic lesions of the liver and allows mapping of lesions, definition of the extent of disease, and determination of relationships to, and involvement of, vascular structures. Ultrasonography is therefore a guide in the choice of operation, with applications from the detection of anatomic variations to the location of intrahepatic vessels in order to be able to occlude them for precise and limited exeresis. This examination technique, with which it is easy to become familiar, does not add any morbidity in itself, as in practice surgical procedures are only slightly prolonged by its inclusion. In future, it should be an indispensable aid to the practice of hepatic surgery as well as to gastrointestinal surgery in general.

3.2 Surgical Anatomy of the Liver

3.2.1 Morphology

The liver is an ovoid, transversely oriented structure that presents a rounded and voluminous right extremity, the left extremity being more slender. Three surfaces can be described:

1. *Superior (Diaphragmatic) Surface* (Figs. 3.1 and 3.2). The curvature of the superior surface matches that of the diaphragm. The insertion of the falciform ligament divides the superior surface into two lobes that are immediately apparent at laparotomy. The insertion of the ligament begins at the superior extremity of the groove for the inferior vena cava on the posterior aspect and continues anteriorly and to the left, to terminate on the anterior border at the level of the ligamentum teres.
2. *Inferior (Visceral) Surface* (Fig. 3.3). This presents several fissures delimiting different lobes. Two anteroposterior fissures are joined by a third transverse fissure (at the hilum), forming the shape of an "H". The left anteroposterior fissure, in the anterior prehilar region, lodges the ligamentum teres (round ligament). The right anteroposterior fissure exists only in the anterior prehilar part and is related to the gallbladder, which is in the cystic fossa. The transverse fissure at the hilum (porta hepatis) connects the two preceding fissures. At the hilum, the structures that constitute the inferior hepatic pedicle, the portal vein, hepatic artery, biliary ducts, nerves, and lymphatic vessels, enter the liver.
3. *Posterior (Diaphragmatic) Surface* (Fig. 3.3). This surface is marked by two vertical grooves. The right groove lodges the inferior vena cava. The large orifices of the hepatic veins are located in the superior part of the groove, being usually the right hepatic vein and a common trunk comprised of the left and middle hepatic veins. However, all along the groove there are very small hepatic veins entering the vena cava. Some of the more voluminous among them come from the caudate lobe. These structures as a whole form the posterior pedicle of the liver. The left groove, which is more restricted, contains the residual fibers of the ligamentum venosum, and is an extension of the groove described on the inferior surface. In the posterior retrohilar region, it lodges the Arantius canal (ligamentum venosum). Three borders are formed between these surfaces:
    1. *Anterior Border.* This is situated at the junction of the superior and inferior surfaces. It forms a sharp, thin edge.
    2. *Posteroinferior Border.* This demarcates the inferior and posterior surfaces of the right lobe. Inferior to the groove of the vena cava, it is directly in contact with the caudate process posterior to the hilum.
    3. *Posterosuperior Border.* This is the junction of the superior and posterior surfaces.

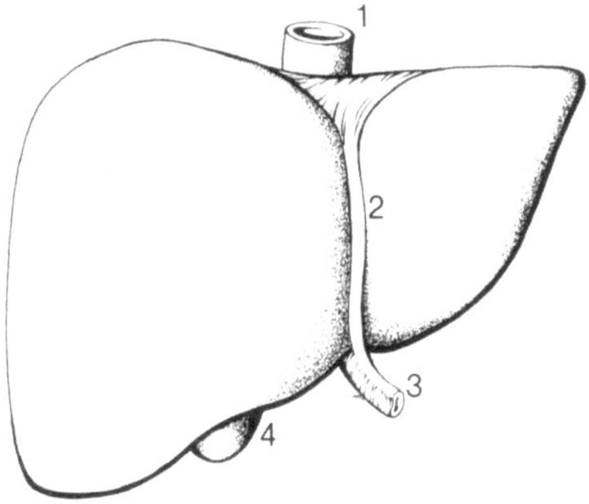

Fig. 3.1. The anterior surface of the liver; *1,* inferior vena cava; *2,* falciform ligament; *3,* ligamentum teres; *4,* gallbladder

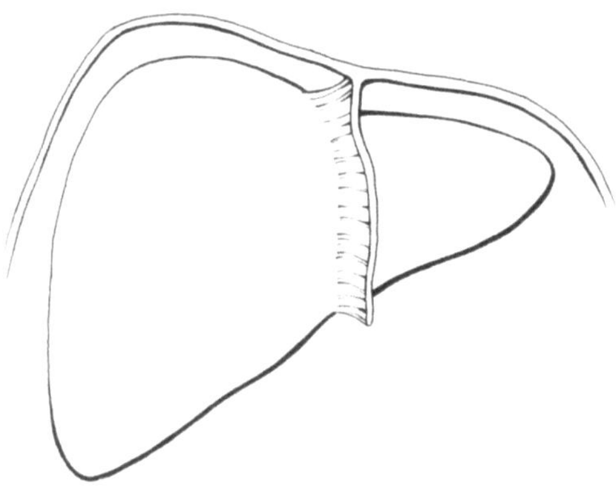

Fig. 3.2. The falciform ligament divides the superior surface of the liver into two parts, the right lobe being located to the right of the ligament, the left lobe to the left of the ligament

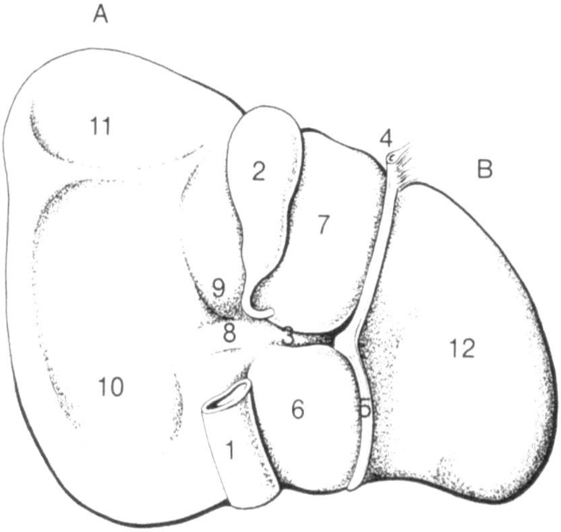

Fig. 3.3. The inferior surface of the liver. *A,* right lobe of the liver. *B,* left lobe of the liver; *1,* inferior vena cava; *2,* gallbladder; *3,* porta hepatis (hilum; transverse fissure of the liver); *4,* ligamentum teres (round ligament); *5,* ligamentum venosus (ductus Arantii); *6,* caudate lobe; *7,* quadrate lobe; *8,* caudate process; *9,* duodenal impression; *10,* renal impression; *11,* colic impression; *12,* gastric impression

The gross structure of the liver is very variable, according to general morphological type (brevilineal or longilineal) because the organ moulds itself to the contours of the diaphragm and surrounding viscera. One type, that develops mainly anteriorly, is ventropetal, and rather flat. Another type, predominantly posterior in development, is squat, thick, and dorsopetal (Figs. 3.4 and 3.5). The transverse variation is the most important one. There are cases in which the liver has developed more laterally, with a large quadrate lobe and a well-developed left lobe occupying part of the left hypochondrium and extending as far as the spleen. The right lobe extends almost to the flank. However, there are variations which extend in a sagittal direction on the right: the right lobe may extend almost to the right iliac fossa, whereas the left lobe barely reaches the midline.

According to Couinaud [16], there is a constant relationship between the distance from the portal bifurcation to the anterior edge of the liver, and the distance from this division to the hepatic veins. If one draws a curved line from the hepatic veins, passing through the hilum at the level of the bifurcation of the portal vein, to the anterior edge of the liver, the portal bifurcation is practically always at the midpoint of this line. The ratio r between the preportal and retroportal segments has one of the highest biometric correlation coefficients ($r = 0.793$; Fig. 3.6).

The liver is surrounded by a fibrous tunic, the capsule of Glisson. This covers the external surface of the organ, encircles the hilum, and is continued into the interior of the organ through ramifications of the hepatic pedicle, for which it forms an enveloping sheath. This vasculobiliary sheath presents a certain number of condensations on the inferior surface of the liver. At the hilum, it becomes the hilar sheath, which is particularly important as it can be detached from the parenchyma without causing any hemorrhage. A second capsular thickening lines the cystic fossa. This is the vesicular sheath. The umbilical sheath forms the floor of the fissure for the ligamentum teres, and the Arantius sheath forms the floor of the fissure for the ligamentum venosum (ductus Arantii). These different formations are in uninterrupted continuity with each other. They ensheath the vasculobiliary elements, and where the latter penetrate the parenchyma, they draw along with them the connective tissue sheath, which forms a perivasculobiliary sheath continuous with the pedicle.

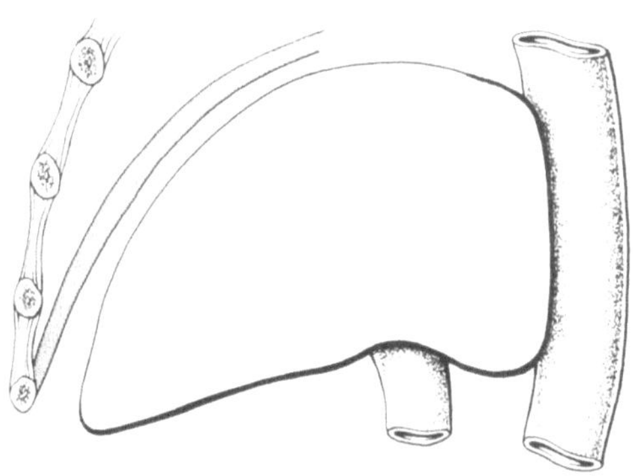

Fig. 3.4. Dorsopetal liver

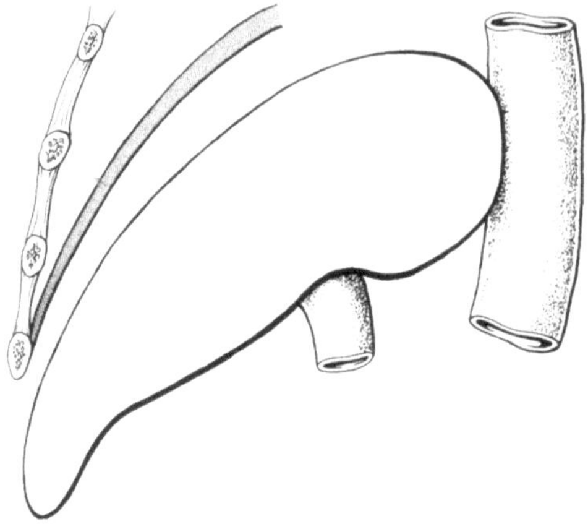

Fig. 3.5. Ventropetal liver

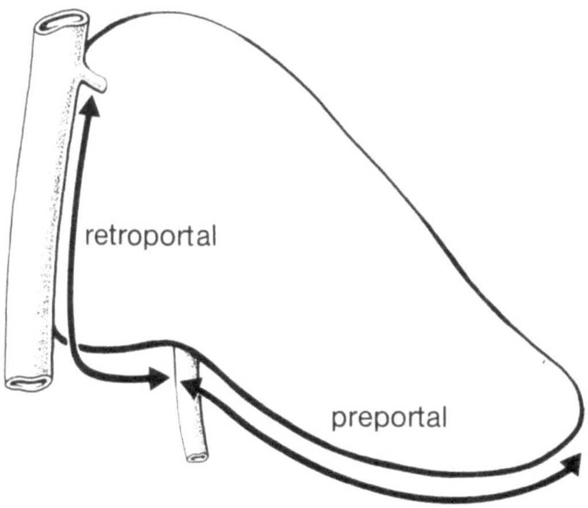

Fig. 3.6. Relationship between the retroportal and the preportal segments of the liver

3.2.2 Supports (Ligaments)

The liver is a fixed organ. Its supports are:

1. The reciprocal pressure of various abdominal viscera.
2. The hepatic ligaments, of which there are three: (a) the lesser omentum, (b) the falciform ligament, and (c) the coronary ligament (right triangular ligament and left triangular ligament).
3. The inferior vena cava, a most important factor because of its intimate attachment to the vertebral column. The liver is connected to it by the hepatic veins.

3.2.3 Relations

The liver is a thoracoabdominal, supramesocolic organ, entirely covered by the thoracic cage, rendering the surgical approach difficult. The relations of the three surfaces of the liver should be considered:

1. *Superior Surface* (Fig. 3.7). Lying just inferior to the diaphragm, the superior surface extends slightly beyond the right costal margin. It crosses the upper epigastric region to extend into the left hypochondrium. Between the abdominal wall and the liver, the peritoneal cavity is divided into the right and left hepato-diaphragmatic recesses by the falciform ligament.
2. *Inferior Surface*. Lodged in the cystic fossa, the gallbladder is directly related to this surface. It is intimately apposed to the liver via the peritoneum and the vessels. With the gallbladder intervening, the liver rests on the supramesocolic viscera. The right lobe is directly related to the right (hepatic) colic flexure, the first part of the duodenum, and the superior pole of the right kidney. The quadrate lobe rests on the lesser omentum and gastric antrum. The left lobe is related to the anterior surface of the stomach. The supramesocolic viscera and the inferior surface of the liver delimit the infrahepatic recess.

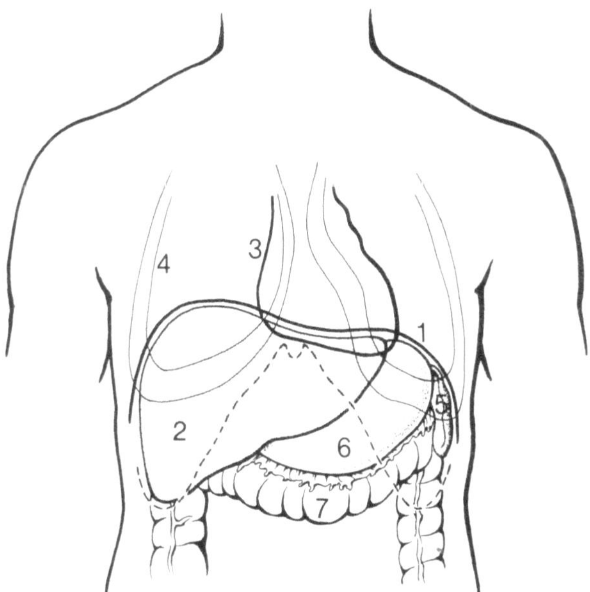

Fig. 3.7. The liver: a thoracoabdominal viscus. *1*, diaphragm; *2*, liver; *3*, heart; *4*, lung; *5*, spleen; *6*, stomach; *7*, colon

3. *Posterior Surface* (Fig. 3.8). This is mostly retroperitoneal. The right lobe covers the right suprarenal gland and the superior pole of the right kidney, and is related to the costodiaphragmatic recess. Posterior to the right triangular ligament, the liver relates directly to the posterior abdominal wall without peritoneal interposition. The important relation of the right lobe is the anterior aspect of the inferior vena cava. The posterior surface of the left lobe is related posteriorly to the anterior aspect of the esophagus.

3.2.4 Functional Anatomy

The intrahepatic vasculature determines the segmentation of the liver. It has been defined by Ton That Tung [54], Couinaud [16], and Lortat-Jacob [29]. The liver has two pedicles, the inferior (hepatic) pedicle, and the posterosuperior pedicle, provided by the hepatic veins. Within the parenchyma, these elements always ramify in the same way, thus allowing the definition of vascular territories: sectors and segments separated by well-defined planes supplied by their own branches.

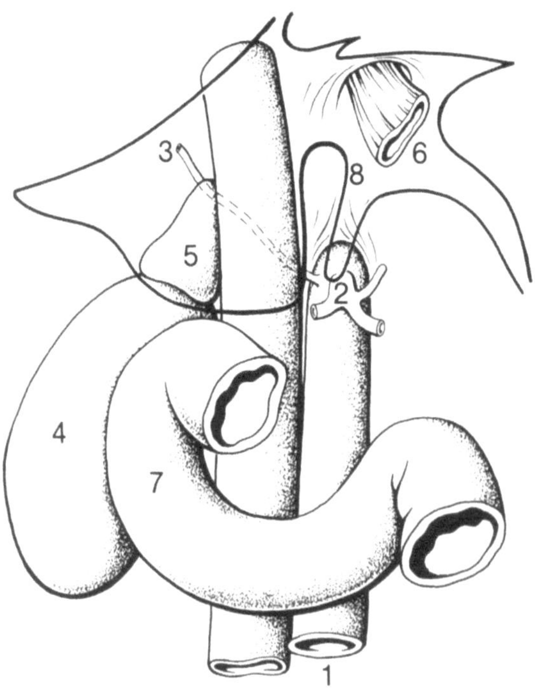

Fig. 3.8. Posterior relations of the liver; *1*, abdominal aorta; *2*, celiac trunk; *3*, right phrenic artery; *4*, right kidney; *5*, right suprarenal gland; *6*, esophagus; *7*, duodenum; *8*, coronary ligament

3.2.4.1 Organization of the Branches of the Portal Pedicle (Figs. 3.9–3.11)

The distributions of the portal vein, the hepatic artery and the intrahepatic biliary ducts are identical, and may be described with reference to the distribution of the portal vein.

Fissures. The principal portal or sagittal fissure separates the right part of the liver from the left. It follows a plane inclined 75° to the inferior surface, and is open to the left. The fissure plane goes through the floor of the cystic fossa, transecting the hilum. Posterosuperiorly, it passes to the left of the inferior vena cava. The right portal fissure divides the right part of the liver into a paramedian sector and a lateral sector. It is less demarcated than the principal fissure. At the anterior border of the liver, it starts at a point equidistant from the right anterolateral angle of the liver and the right border of the cystic fossa. On the inferior surface, it follows a line that runs from this point to the right part of the hilum. On the superior surface, it ends at the junction of the right hepatic vein and the inferior vena cava. The left portal fissure divides the left part of the liver into a left lateral sector and a left paramedian sector. It runs transversely to join the posterior extremity of the fissure for the ligamentum teres. The portal fissures thus delimit the hepatic sectors irrigated by the branches of the portal vein and drained by the hepatic veins that fill in the fissure planes. The pattern of portal vascularization within these sectors permits the distinction of segments. Within a sector, the separation planes between portal segments do not strictly apply to the hepatic veins.

Territories. On the right, the paramedian sector is divided into two segments, the right anterior paramedian segment (V), and the right posterior paramedian segment (VIII). The right lateral sector is divided into the right anterior lateral segment (VI) and the right posterior lateral segment (VII). The latter segment has a very posterior and inferior position, and forms the base of segment VIII. The transverse separation plane between the anterior and posterior segments is perpendicular to the right hepatic vein.

On the left, the left paramedian sector is divided into the anterior (III) and posterior (IV) segments by the fissure for the ligamentum teres. This corresponds to the fissure which separates the left lobe from the quadrate lobe. Segment IV is larger than the classical quadrate lobe. It is entirely located anterior to the hilum, and extends from the principal portal fissure to the fissure for the ligamentum teres. On the superior surface, it encompasses the hilum and occupies the whole zone situated between the principal fissure on the right and the insertion of the falciform ligament on the left. Posteriorly, it covers the dorsal sector (caudate lobe).

The left lateral paramedian sector (III) forms the major part of the superior face of the left lobe and the anterior half of the inferior face. The left lateral sector consists only of segment II covered superiorly and anteriorly by segment III. The dorsal sector (caudate lobe) forms segment I. It is delimited by the posterior portal fissure. On the right, the fissure is occupied by the inferior vena cava and is prolonged by the caudate process, toward the hilum. On the left, it is the prolongation of the fissure for the ligamentum teres: the fissure for the ligamentum venosum. Concerning its vascularization, segment I belongs to the left lobe of the liver rather than to the right.

Organization

Portal Vein. This vein (Fig. 3.9) is the largest and most posterior element of the hepatic pedicle. It is bifurcated at an angle of approximately 120°. The left trunk is twice as long and twice as thin as the right (3-5 cm long in the section traversing the hilum). The left branch, inclined anteriorly at an angle of 100°, forms the umbilical recess of Rex in an anteroposterior position within the fissure for the ligamentum teres. It terminates as two branches, one for segments III and IV, and one for segment II. The branch supplying segment III arises from the left horn of the umbilical recess; the branch to segment IV originates in the right horn. The vein of segment II (lateral vein or left posterior angular vein) runs almost horizontally.

The left trunk, in its initial portion, provides segment I with some collateral veins. Hence, the branches to segments III and IV have an ascending recurrent course that is in a much more superficial plane than the left branch of the portal vein. Furthermore, it is crossed anteriorly by the vein of segment IV.

The distribution of the right branch of the portal vein is more variable than that of the left branch. The right branch is comparatively squat, and measures 2 cm in the hilum. In its hilar course it provides some branches to segment I. It continues the course of the portal trunk for 1-3 cm before two terminal branches arise: the right paramedian vein and the right lateral vein. The right paramedian vein initially takes a sagittal posteroanterior course, then becomes anteroposterior and describes a curve that is concave superiorly and posteriorly. It ends in two or more branches. The anterior and inferior collateral veins are distributed to segment V, the posterior and superior ones to segment VIII. The right lateral vein continues the course of the right portal vein for 1 cm and curves posteriorly, superiorly, and medially in the direction of the right hepatic vein. It seems to follow the curve of the right hepatic border. Segment VI receives branches from the convex and horizontal portion of the right branch of the portal vein. Segment VII is very voluminous, and is irrigated by the terminal branches of the right lateral vein.

Hepatic Artery. Understanding of the surgical anatomy of the hepatic artery has benefited considerably from the work of Michels [38] and Mellière [36]. The classical disposition (present in only 60% of cases) is a single hepatic artery arising from the celiac (hepatosplenic) trunk. This single artery divides inferior to the hilum, to the left of the main fissure, into a branch to the left lobe of the liver and a branch to the right lobe.

In 40% of cases, this arrangement is not present. There may be three hepatic arteries: a hepatic artery arising from the celiac trunk (median hepatic artery), a right hepatic artery arising from the superior mesenteric artery, and a left hepatic artery arising from the left gastric artery. Within the liver, the hepatic arteries follow the branches of the portal vein, generally with the branches in hypoportal position. They are enclosed in a thick sheath, which is the continuation of the capsula hepatitis.

Intrahepatic Biliary Ducts. These follow the distribution of the portal venous branches and are generally in epiportal positions, unlike the arteries. The junction of the two main right and left extrahepatic branches defines the superior biliary confluence.

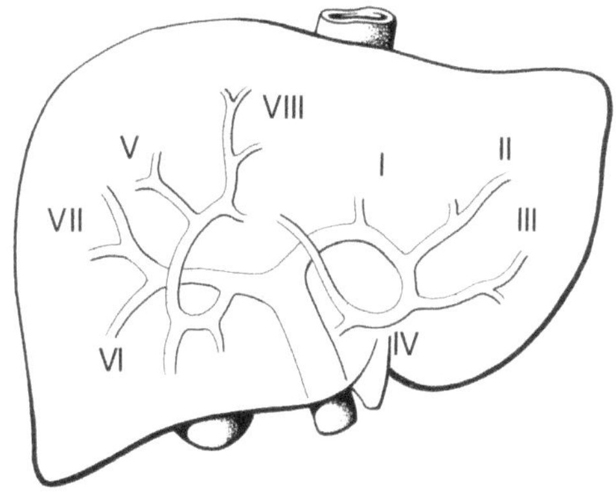

Fig. 3.9. Branches of the portal vein; classical arrangement, anterior view; segments are indicated by *roman numerals*

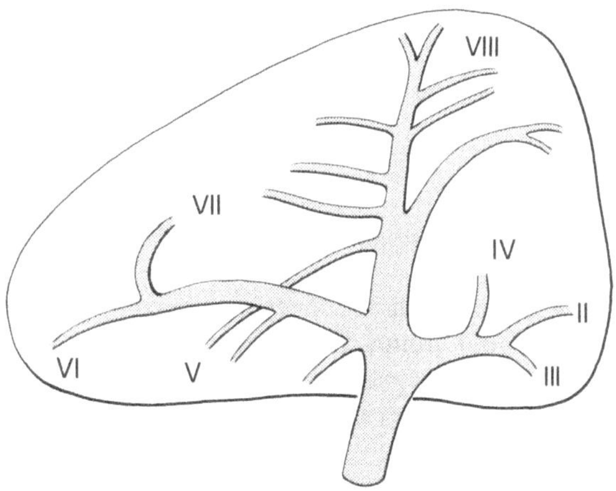

Fig. 3.10. Branches of the portal vein; right lateral view of a portal phlebogram; segments are indicated by *roman numerals* (according to Ton That Tung [55])

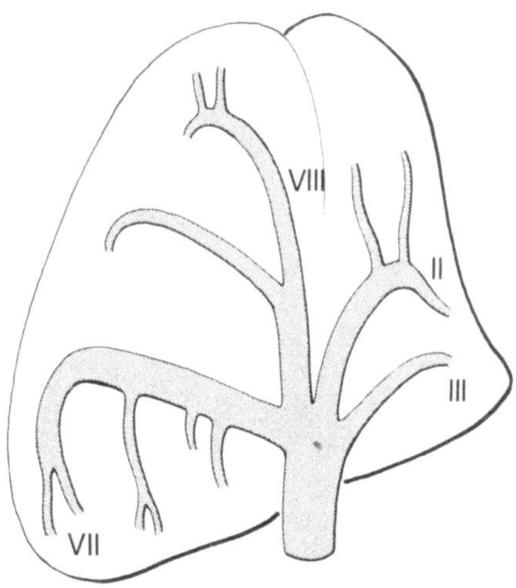

Fig. 3.11. Intrahepatic biliary ducts; right lateral view of an intrahepatic cholangiogram; segments are indicated by *roman numerals* (according to Ton That Tung [55])

In the right lobe of the liver, the biliary drainage of the lateral sector is effected through the right lateral duct for segments VI and VII, and for segments V and VIII through the right paramedian duct. The lateral duct passes directly posterior to the right paramedian vein. It is joined by the right paramedian duct to form the right hepatic duct superior and anterior to the right branch of the portal vein.

In the left lobe of the liver, the ducts of segments II and III flow together to form the left hepatic duct on the left portal fissure. Several small ducts that drain segment IV form a single trunk which flows into the horizontal portion of the left hepatic duct. The dorsal sector (segment I) is drained to both the right and left by several ductules.

The right and left hepatic ducts flow together into the hilum, anterior to the proximal part of the right branch of the portal vein. The convergence occurs superior to and to the right of the arterial division. The angle formed by the two ducts is 80°. The right hepatic duct continues as the common hepatic duct. Variations are very frequent. Rarely, the right and left ducts are absent, and the sectorial ducts form the convergence directly. The right hepatic duct is absent in 40% of cases. Both the right sectorial ducts may flow together into the left branch. Alternatively, a right sectorial duct may enter the hepatic duct or the left branch separately.

3.2.4.2 Organization of Hepatic Veins (Fig. 3.12)

The efferent pedicle conveying blood from the liver to the inferior vena cava consists of four groups of hepatic veins:

1. The dorsal veins come from the caudate lobe and flow directly into the inferior vena cava. They define a dorsal hepatic sector coinciding with the dorsal portal sector.

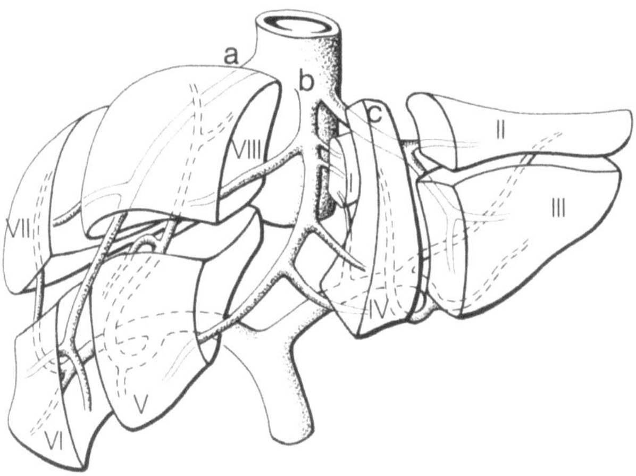

Fig. 3.12. Hepatic veins; *a*, right hepatic vein; *b*, middle hepatic vein; *c*, left hepatic vein; segments are indicated by *roman numerals*

2. The left hepatic vein is situated in the left fissural plane. It drains only the classical left lobe of the liver (segments II and III). It is enclosed superiorly and anteriorly by segment II, and inferiorly and posteriorly it rests on segment III. The left hepatic vein follows the posterior border of the liver and ends in a common trunk with the middle hepatic vein.
3. The middle hepatic vein, or sagittal vein, is superficial anteriorly, and lies within the plane between the right and left parts. It comes close to the inferior surface deep to the cystic fossa. It drains the right paramedian sector (segments V and VIII) and segment IV of the left part of the liver. Usually segment V is drained by its own vein. A voluminous vein frequently enters the sagittal vein from the superior aspect and serves segment VIII. Two veins drain segment IV. The middle hepatic vein joins the inferior vena cava by a common trunk with the left hepatic vein. The opening to the vena cava is set at an angle of approximately 60°.
4. The right hepatic vein is the largest of the four veins. It divides the paramedian sector from the right lateral sector and drains mainly the right lateral sector (segments VI and VII). It arises from two branches that drain segment VI and passes anterior to the right branch of the portal vein. It is then covered, anteriorly and above all laterally, by the voluminous segment VII, from which numerous veins join the right hepatic vein at an acute angle. The posterior veins of segment VII join the right hepatic vein near its opening into the inferior vena cava. This opening, on the right anterior side of the inferior vena cava is set at an angle of 45°.

3.2.5 Lymphatic Vessels and Nerves

There are two lymphatic chains in the portal pedicle: one associated with the biliary duct, the other with the artery. They drain into both the great right and left lymphatic channels of the abdomen. Through the diaphragm and posteriorly, some of the hepatic lymph reaches the thorax directly. The volume of the lymphatic drainage of the liver is particularly significant, and reflects the portal pressure. Branches of the celiac plexus, the celiac ganglia, and the vagus nerve, form the hepatic plexus, which is itself divided into the anterior plexus and the posterior plexus.

3.2.6 Atlas of Sonographic Anatomical Sections (Figs. 3.13–3.22) (from Senecail et al. [48])

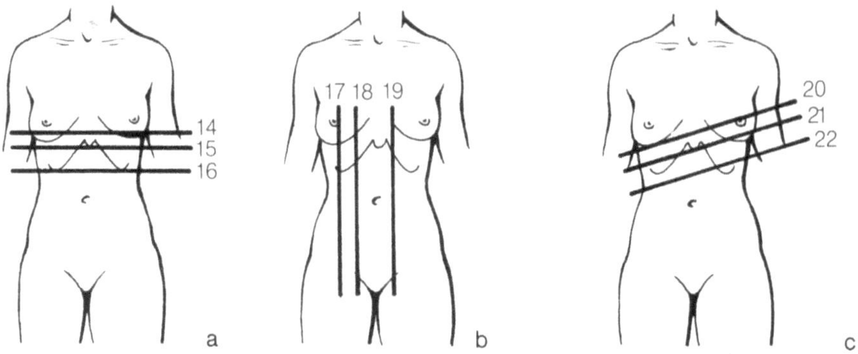

Fig. 3.13 a–c. Relationship between sonography and anatomy of the liver. **a** 3 horizontal sections; the *planes of section* indicated by *numbers 14–16* are illustrated in Figs. 3.14–16, respectively. **b** 3 sagittal sections; the *planes of section* indicated by *numbers 17–19* are illustrated in Figs. 3.17–19, respectively. **c** 3 oblique sections; the *planes of section* indicated by *numbers 20–22* are illustrated in Figs. 3.20–22, respectively

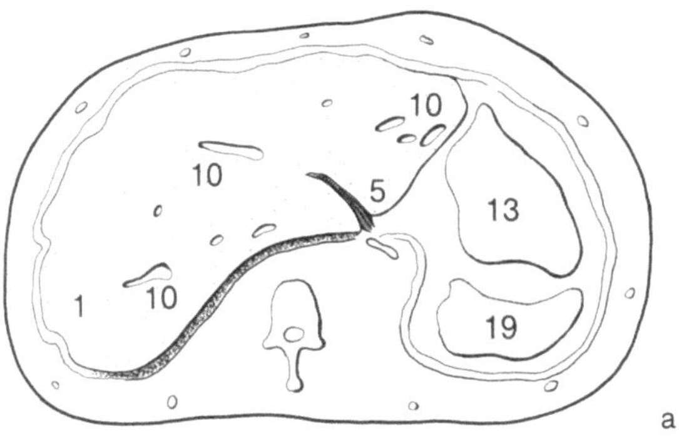

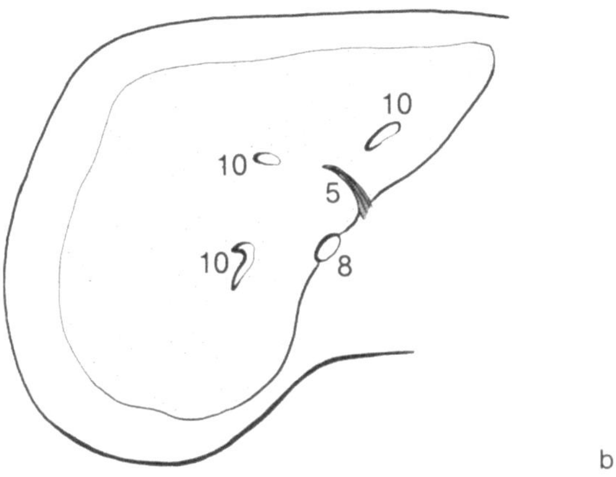

Fig. 3.14 a, b. Transverse section, upper level shown in Fig. 3.13 a. **a** Cadaver; *1,* right lobe of liver; *5,* ligamentum venosum; *10,* hepatic veins; *13,* stomach; *19,* spleen. **b** Sonogram; *8,* inferior vena cava

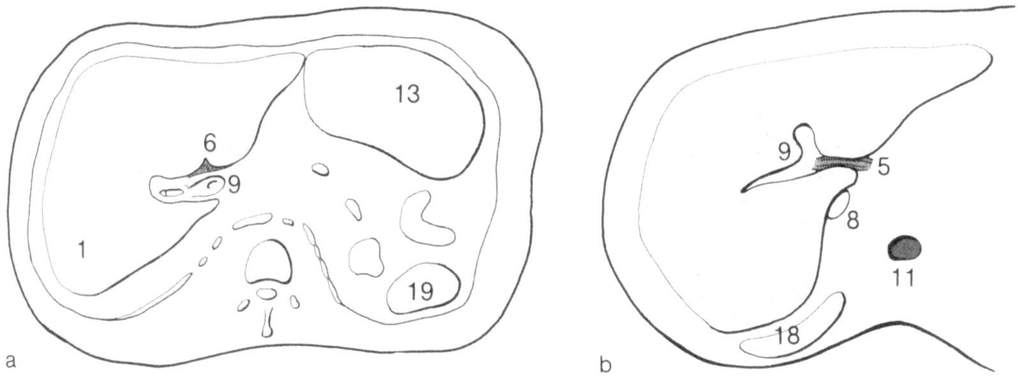

Fig. 3.15 a, b. Transverse section, middle level shown in Fig. 3.13 a. **a** Cadaver; *1,* right lobe of liver; *6,* ligamentum teres; *9,* portal vein; *13,* stomach; *19,* spleen. **b** Sonogram; *5,* ligamentum venosum; *8,* inferior vena cava; *11,* abdominal aorta; *18,* right suprarenal gland

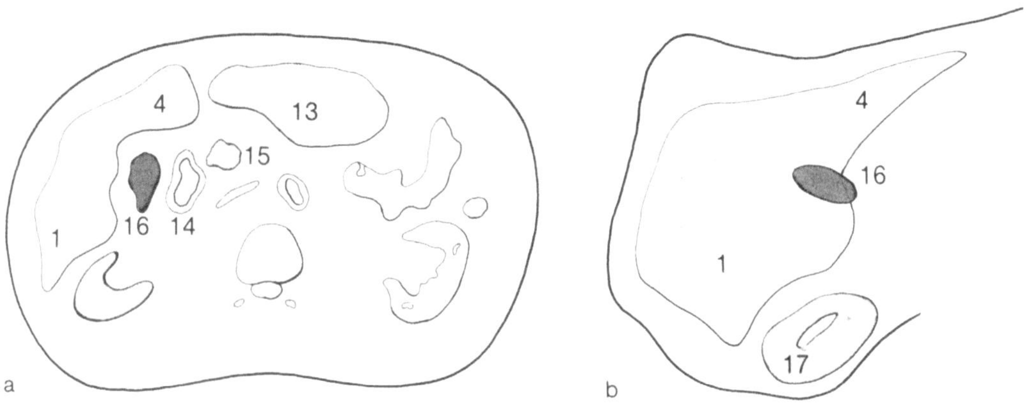

Fig. 3.16 a, b. Transverse section, lower level shown in Fig. 3.13 a. **a** Cadaver; *1,* right lobe of liver; *4,* quadrate lobe; *13,* stomach; *14,* duodenum; *15,* pancreas; *16,* gallbladder. **b** Sonogram; *17,* right kidney.

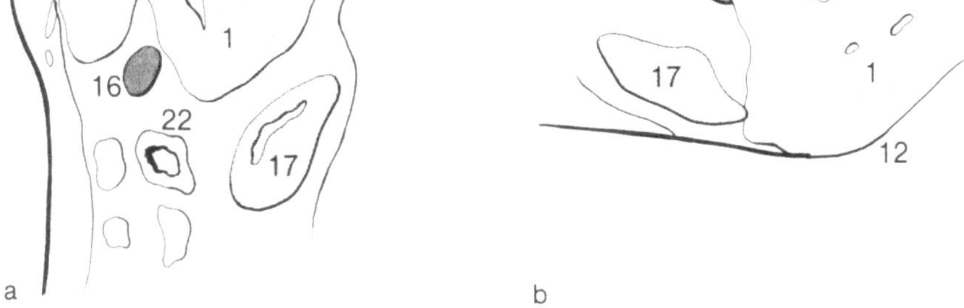

Fig. 3.17 a, b. Right lateral section shown in Fig. 3.13 b. **a** Cadaver; *1,* right lobe of liver; *16,* gallbladder; *17,* right kidney; *22,* colon. **b** Sonogram; *9,* portal vein; *12,* diaphragm

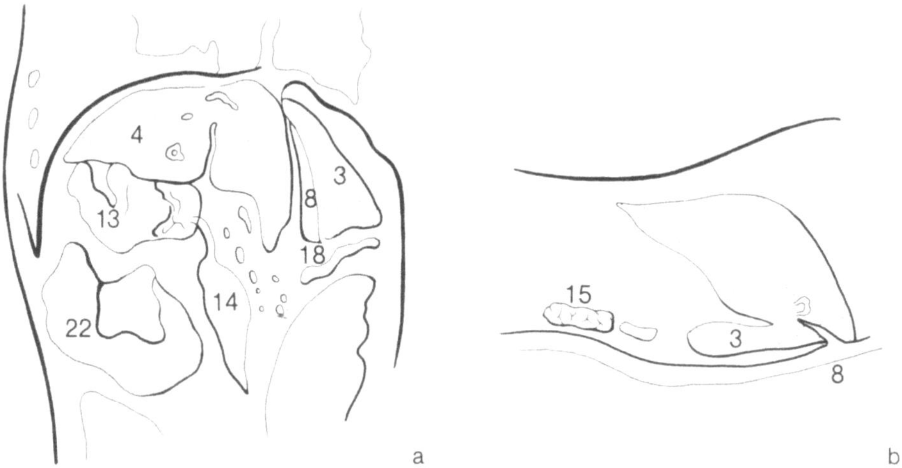

Fig. 3.18 a, b. Right paramedian sagittal section shown in Fig. 3.13 b. **a** Cadaver; *3*, caudate lobe; *4*, quadrate lobe; *8*, inferior vena cava; *13*, stomach; *14*, duodenum; *18*, right suprarenal gland; *22*, colon. **b** Sonogram; *15*, pancreas

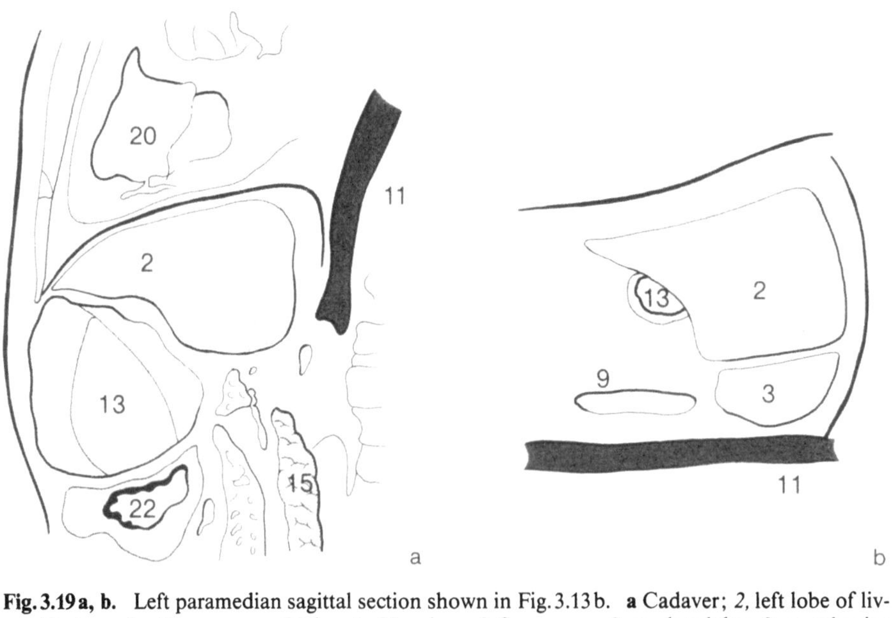

Fig. 3.19 a, b. Left paramedian sagittal section shown in Fig. 3.13 b. **a** Cadaver; *2*, left lobe of liver; *13*, stomach; *15*, pancreas; *20*, heart; *22*, colon. **b** Sonogram; *3*, caudate lobe; *9*, portal vein; *11*, abdominal aorta

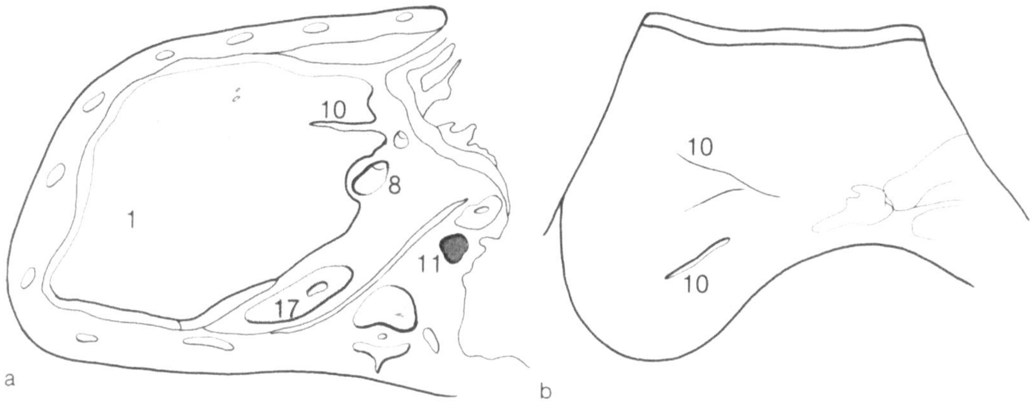

Fig. 3.20 a, b. Oblique section, upper level shown in Fig. 3.13 c. **a** Cadaver; *1,* right lobe of liver; *8,* inferior vena cava; *10,* hepatic veins; *11,* abdominal aorta; *17,* right kidney; *21,* right side of diaphragm. **b** Sonogram

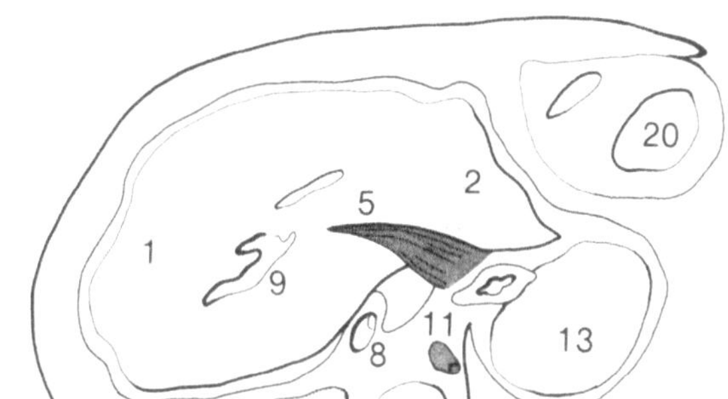

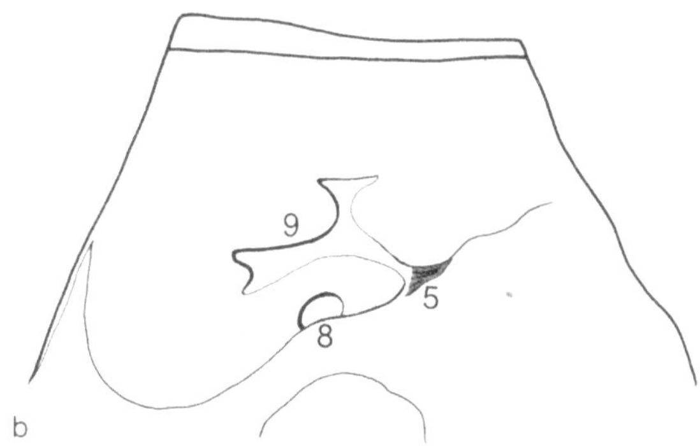

Fig. 3.21 a, b. Oblique section, middle level shown in Fig. 3.13 c. **a** Cadaver; *1,* right lobe of liver; *2,* left lobe of liver; *5,* ligamentum venosum; *8,* inferior vena cava; *9,* portal vein; *11,* abdominal aorta; *13,* stomach; *17,* right kidney; *20,* heart. **b** Sonogram

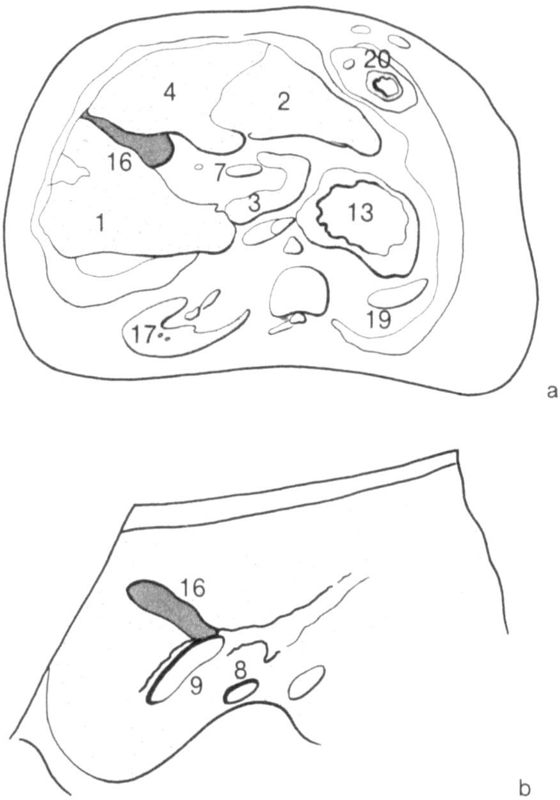

Fig. 3.22 a, b. Oblique section, lower level shown in Fig. 3.13 c. **a** Cadaver; *1,* right lobe of liver; *2,* left lobe of liver; *3,* caudate lobe; *4,* quadrate lobe; *7,* porta hepatis (hilum); *13,* stomach; *16,* gallbladder; *17,* right kidney; *19,* spleen; *20,* colon. **b** Sonogram; *8,* inferior vena cava; *9,* portal vein

3.3 Analytical Study

3.3.1 Technical Difficulties

Several difficulties may be encountered in hepatic ultrasonography:

1. Approach. Any surgical approach allows the utilization of hepatic ultrasonography, as long as it is possible to slip a probe between the liver and the diaphragm. Only significant adhesion can impede its implementation, if the approach used precludes adhesiotomy [9].

2. Morphotype. According to Duvauferrier [17], the morphotype of the subject [49] is responsible for 8% of the failures in conventional ultrasonography, whereas it does not interfere with intraoperative ultrasonography.

3. The Attachments of the Liver. The superior surface of the liver is the most suitable one for sonography, so it may be very useful to section the *ligamentum teres* and the *falciform ligament* as far posteriorly as possible. Section of the *triangular ligaments* is not useful in itself.

4. Surface Irregularities. The sonographic exploration of a cirrhotic liver can be particularly difficult due to surface irregularities. The existence of more or less pronounced hobnail-like protuberances and pit-like depressions can make contact between the probe and the organ difficult. In such cases, a special convex probe can be used. A water bag can also be interposed between the probe and the liver surface.

5. Difficulties in Stereospatial Representation of Hepatic Segments. Difficulty arises from the terminology used for the hepatic sectors and segments, especially the French system of nomenclature. As a matter of fact, this terminology does not take into consideration the liver's topography in situ. Without questioning Couinaud's [16] established systematization, which has been used throughout this study, it is important to point out the works of Agoussou-Voyème [5] and Flament et al. [18] which facilitate the comprehension of certain sonographic images obtained in the study of the liver. These authors point out the anterolateral position of the right paramedian sector (V and VIII) and the posterior position of the right lateral sector (VI and VII).

6. Acoustic Coupling. The use of sterile contact gel is not necessary. The natural moisture of the liver is sufficient [45]. Nonetheless, we make a habit of working in a humid atmosphere by pouring physiological saline solution into the field of operation.

7. The Blind Zone. This is located at the point of immediate contact with the probe, where a 5-mm-thick zone is not explored during ultrasonography. In order to compensate for this inconvenience, the operator may place the probe on the opposite surface (on the inferior surface for superficial lesions of the superior surface) or interpose a sterile glove or waterbag filled with saline between the probe and the hepatic surface.

8. Mobilization of the Probe. Exploration must be carried out gently. Displacement of the probe should be slow and, above all, performed without any excessive pressure. Even moderate pressure on the organ erases the vascular formations which are indispensable landmarks for exploration. This phenomenon occurs prominently when the probe is slipped between the liver and the right lateral wall of the abdomen. In order to avoid any compression of the liver, the probe can be manipulated via movement of its cable.

3.3.2 General Sonographic Properties of the Elements Explored

Hepatic Parenchyma. The parenchymal echostructure of the liver is regular, the even distribution of fine echoes giving the image considerable homogeneity. The occasional heterogeneities observed are due to the multiple vascular sections [51, 56]. As will be shown later, it is less echogenic than the pancreatic parenchyma.

Hepatic Veins. The branches of the *hepatic veins* have smooth walls directly related to and intimately adhering to the hepatic parenchyma [22]. These veins are easily recognizable because they yield perfectly anechogenic, classical images and do not have their own walls, unlike the *portal branches* [33]. In longitudinal section, a vessel appears as an anechogenic layer within the hepatic parenchyma. In transverse or oblique section, the vascular lumen appears as an anechogenic rounded or oval image. It is notable that a distinct, clearly echogenic image of a wall may appear. This boundary image depends on the angle at which the ultrasound beam approaches the hepatic vein; the more perpendicular to the vessels the angle is, the sharper the image is, as Fig. 3.23 shows [17, 56].

Portal Veins. These form with the arterial and biliary elements a true sonographic group. The characteristic sonographic feature of these structures, by which they may be recognized, is the existence of a hyperechogenic surrounding halo that is obvious within the hepatic parenchyma, when compared with the *hepatic veins* [22].

The image is effectively composed of the anechogenic lumen of the venous element, in association with the echoes from the vein wall and satellite echoes from the hepatic artery wall and the biliary duct, as well as echoes coming from the connective tissue of the capsule [17, 28, 33], as Fig. 3.24 demonstrates.

In practice, the vein is identified within this complex image because of its anechogenic lumen and its volume. The artery is identified because of its pulsations. In contrast, the biliary element, in the absence of dilation, is usually identified on the basis of deduction, as is generally situated in an epiportal position.

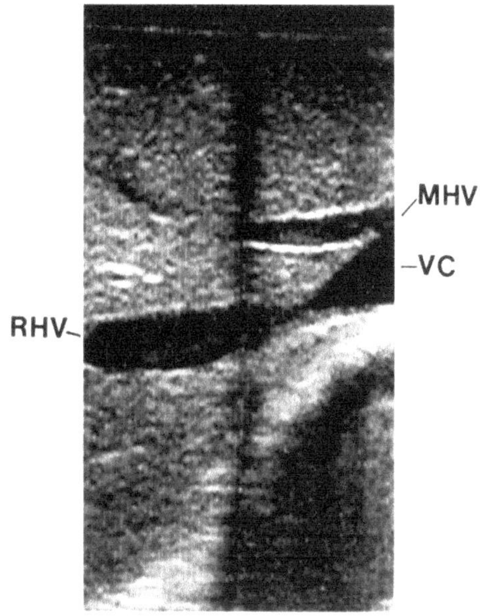

Fig. 3.23. The margin of the middle hepatic vein (*MHV*). The ultrasound beam is perpendicular to the vein. *RHV*, right hepatic vein

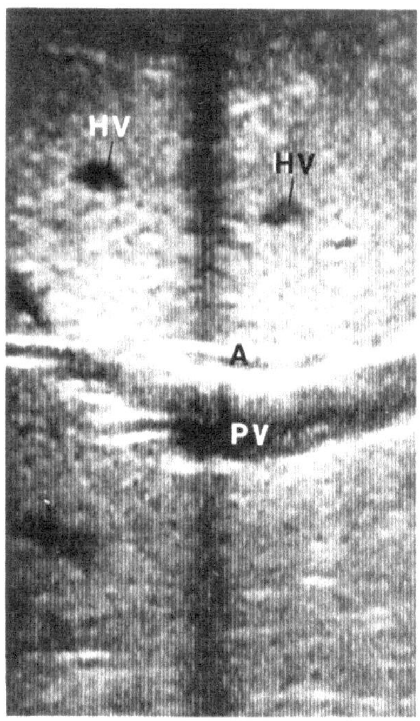

Fig. 3.24. Hyperechogenicity of the margin of portal vein compared with the hepatic vein (*HV*). (PV), portal vein; *A*, artery

Ligaments and Grooves. These structures have been particularly well studied by Sexton and Zehan [50]. They are distinguishable because of their hyperechogenicity. This is notably the case for the ligamentum teres hepatis and the fissure for the ligamentum venosum (Fig. 3.25).

Inferior Vena Cava. According to the beam's incidence, the vena cava may appear as an anechogenic retrohepatic layer, or as a rounded anechogenic formation (Figs. 3.25 and 3.26). It is easily recognized because of the variations in its diameter, which changes with respiration. It may even appear to pulsate, due to pulsation directly transmitted from the right atrium [56]. Finally, fine echoes can be seen moving in the lumen of the vein. These correspond to the circulating blood elements.

3.3.3 Sonographic Guidance

Preliminaries. This chapter will enable the sonographer to become acquainted with the different sonographic sections necessary for recognition of intraparenchymatous formations whose echostructure has already been mentioned. To this purpose, we have selected different easily reproducible sections. Before starting this chapter, the reader should know that:

1. The images have been obtained by placing the probe on the superior surface of the liver.
2. The position of the probe cannot be indicated with millimetric precision, and may need to be varied to obtain the same image from different individuals.

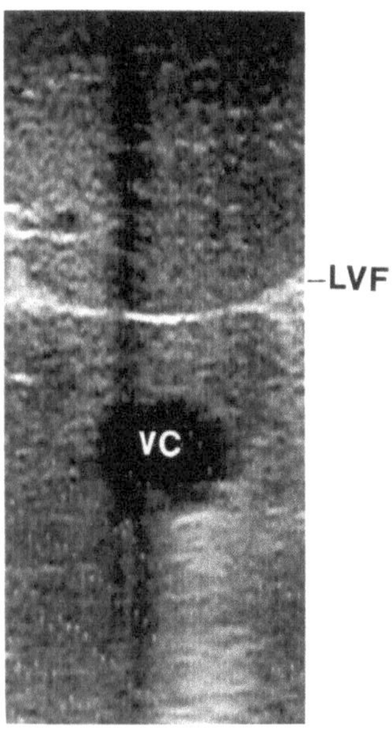

Fig. 3.25. Transverse section of the vena cava, which appears as a round hypoechogenic formation. The hyperechogenicity of the fissure for the ligamentum venosum (*LVF*) delimiting segments I and II is shown. *VC*, vena cava

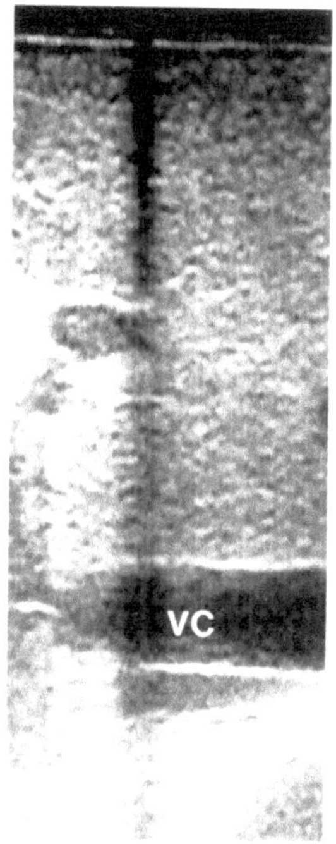

Fig. 3.26. Longitudinal section. The vena cava (*VC*) is seen as a wide hypoechogenic layer. During examination, fine circulating echoes and the pulsations of the vein are seen. Note also the homogeneity of the hepatic parenchyma

3. The orientation of the ultrasound beam is as important as the position of the probe; certain sections have been obtained by simply modifying the orientation of the ultrasound beam.
4. There are two types of section: transverse, and longitudinal.
5. With transverse sections, the right side of the sonogram corresponds to the left side of the organ.
6. With longitudinal sections, the right side of the image corresponds to the posterior part of the organ.

At the end of this chapter, the reader should be capable of recognizing the various vascular elements and also the different hepatic segments, on the basis of Couinaud's system of segmentation [16]. To make this guide easy to assimilate, two views of the liver: frontal and lateral (Figs. 3.27 and 3.28) were performed in order to recreate the spatial configuration of the organ.

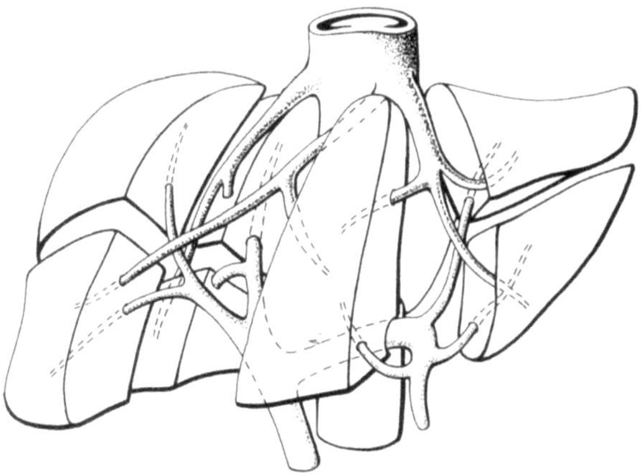

Fig. 3.27. Anterior view of liver

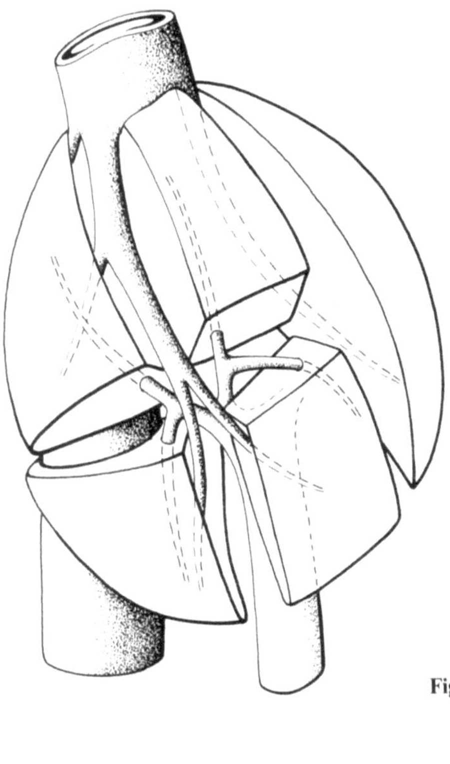

Fig. 3.28. Right lateral view of liver

Methodology. Sonographic exploration of the liver has to be carried out rigorously (Figs. 3.29-3.38). It can be analyzed from three examinations:

1. Identification of the vascular elements, in order to identify the different fissures on the hepatic surface, should be performed initially. Recognition and characterization of the topography of each hepatic segment follows.
2. The second step is detection of hepatic lesions, and characterization of the size, location within the different hepatic segments, number, and relationship to the vascular elements of any such lesions. This may include the investigation of possible vascular invasion or thrombosis, and also the recognition of the vascular pedicle which supplies a tumor.

These two preliminary examinations must be effected slowly, without excessive pressure on the organ, maintaining the sharpness of the image obtained. It may be necessary to remoisten the hepatic surface with saline solution. It may also be necessary to modify the gain; as mentioned above, some appliances are equipped with global, proximal, and distal gain adjustments. The sonographer must monitor the sharpness of the image. It should also be mentioned that the transience of certain images is the result of excessively abrupt mobilization of the probe, which changes the plane of section. This may also be associated with erasure of vessels, above all hepatic veins, due to respiratory movements. In this case one must not modify the position of the probe, but reduce the pressure on the organ.

3. The third step is to perform a sonographically guided puncture biopsy. For this purpose, some probes in the shape of a "T" have a central orifice, which is the case with the probe we use. The puncture needle is introduced through this orifice. Other probes have an adaptable system at the extremity to permit the introduction of the needle. Such mechanisms, although not indispensable, can facilitate manipulations during the technical training period.

   Whatever type of probe is used, the puncture technique is simple: with one hand the surgeon holds the probe, while the other hand introduces the needle. The needle is easily located by its echo, which is displaced at the same time as the needle is moved.

   During the training time, this examination can take longer than 30 min. This interval helps the surgeon to become familiar with sonographic anatomy and the technique. After the initiation time, the examination takes 10 to 15 min.

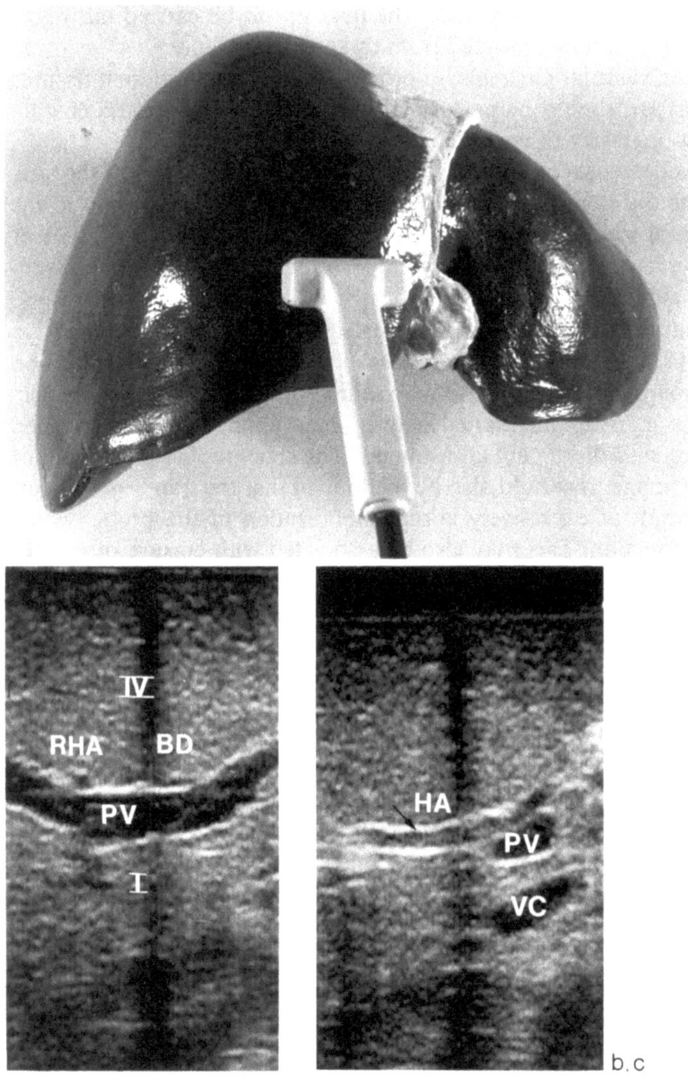

a

b, c

Fig. 3.29 a–c. Transverse section 1: portal bifurcation. **a** Position of the probe. **b** Sonogram; *PV*, portal vein; *RHA*, right hepatic artery; *BD*, bile duct; *I*, segment I; *IV*, segment IV. **c** Variation of the preceding section; image obtained by modifying the position of the ultrasound beam or displacing the probe toward the anterior outline of the liver; *PV*, portal vein; *HA*, division of hepatic artery; *VC*, vena cava

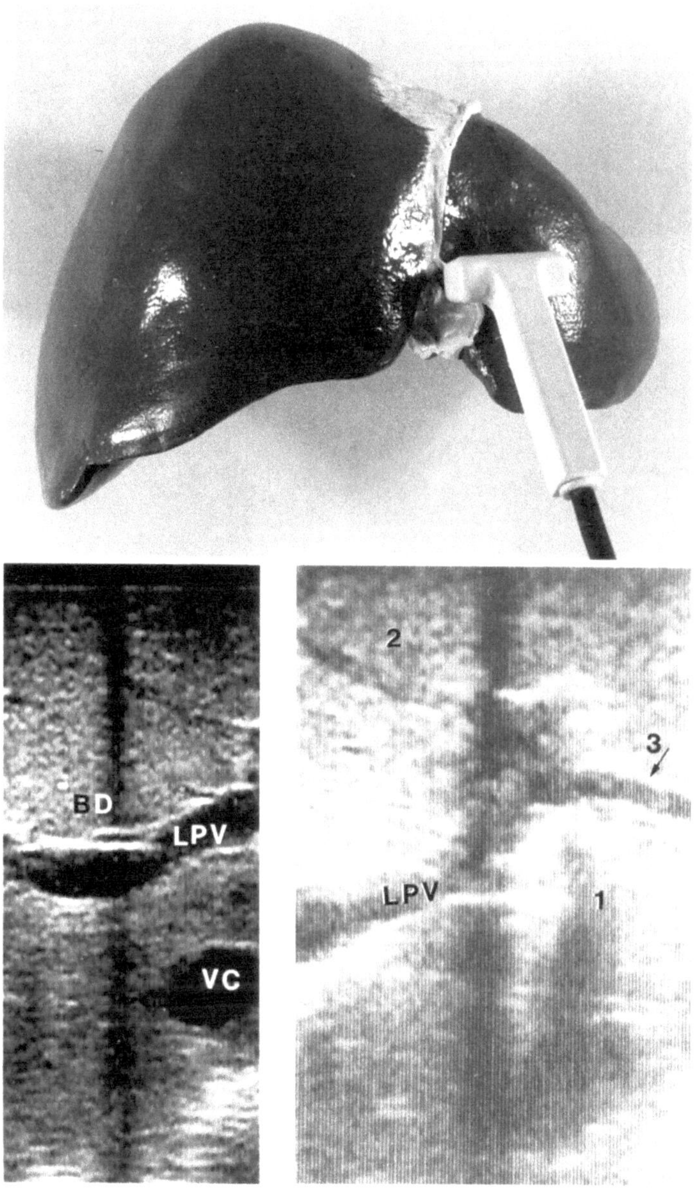

Fig. 3.30 a–c. Transverse section 2: left portal vein. **a** Position of the probe. Starting from section 1, the probe is slowly displaced toward the left, while the ultrasound beam is maintained slightly oblique. **b** Sonogram; *LPV*, left portal vein; *BD*, bile duct; *VC*, vena cava. **c** Sonogram; *1*, portal branch to segment II; *2*, portal branch to segment IV; *LPV*, left portal vein; *3*, portal branch to segment III

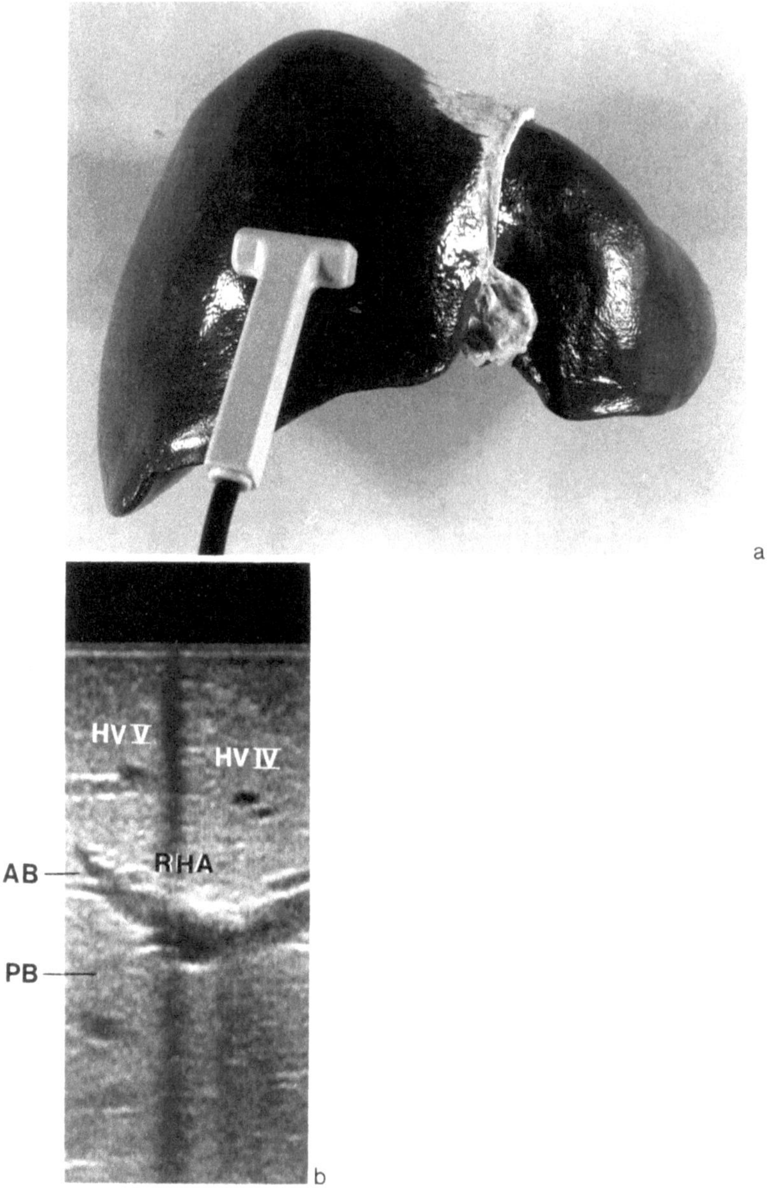

Fig. 3.31 a, b. Transverse section 3: right portal vein. **a** Position of the probe. Starting from the position in section I, the probe is slowly displaced toward the right. The beam's orientation is dependent on the anatomic conditions. **b** Sonogram; *AB,* anterior branch of right portal vein; *PB,* posterior branch of right portal vein; *RHA,* right hepatic artery; *HV V,* hepatic vein draining segment V; *HV IV,* hepatic vein draining segment IV. It is possible, by slowly displacing the probe backwards, i.e., toward the vena cava, to register the confluence of both hepatic veins to form the middle hepatic vein

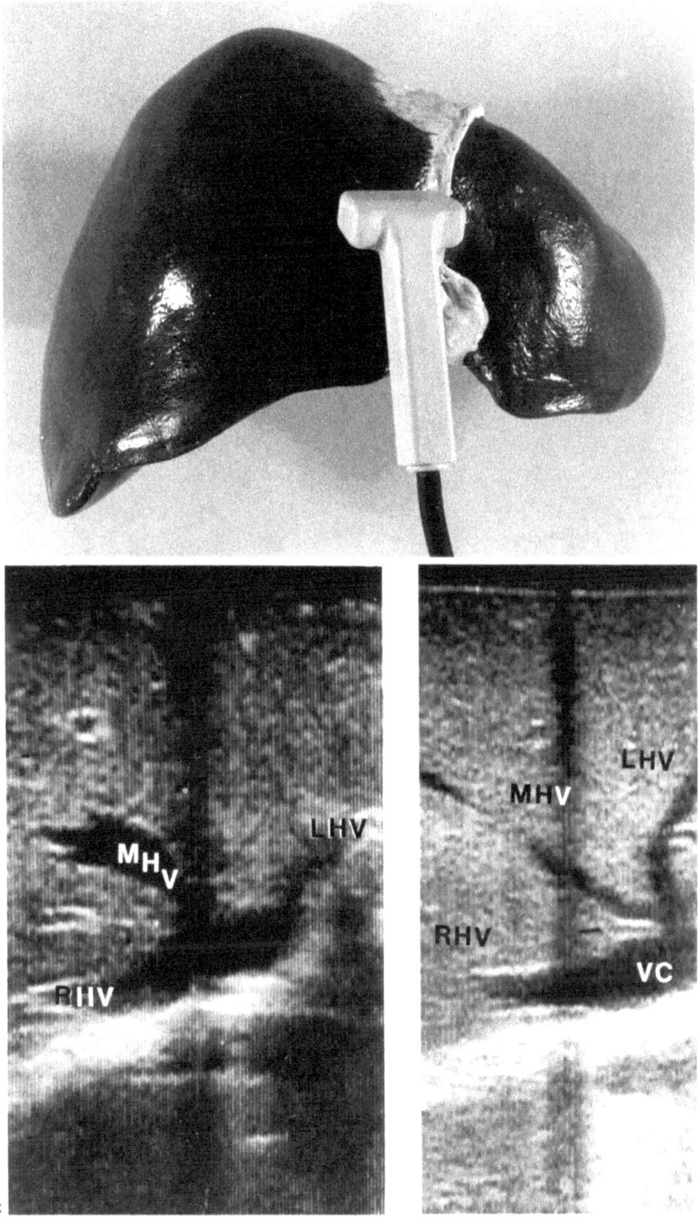

Fig. 3.32 a–c. Transverse section 4: openings of hepatic veins. **a** Position of the probe. The probe is placed approximately halfway between the anterior edge of the liver and the inferior vena cava. Here, the beam will always be very recurrent. To effect this section, especially if the probe is voluminous, the sonographer must take care not to compress the parenchyma, to avoid erasing vascular formations. **b** Sonogram. This section obtains the classical trident image with three hepatic veins: *RHV,* right hepatic vein; *MHV,* middle hepatic vein; *LHV,* left hepatic vein. The left and the middle hepatic veins have no common trunk. **c** Sonogram showing the hepatic veins, left and middle, presenting a common trunk, the classical arrangement; *VC,* vena cava.

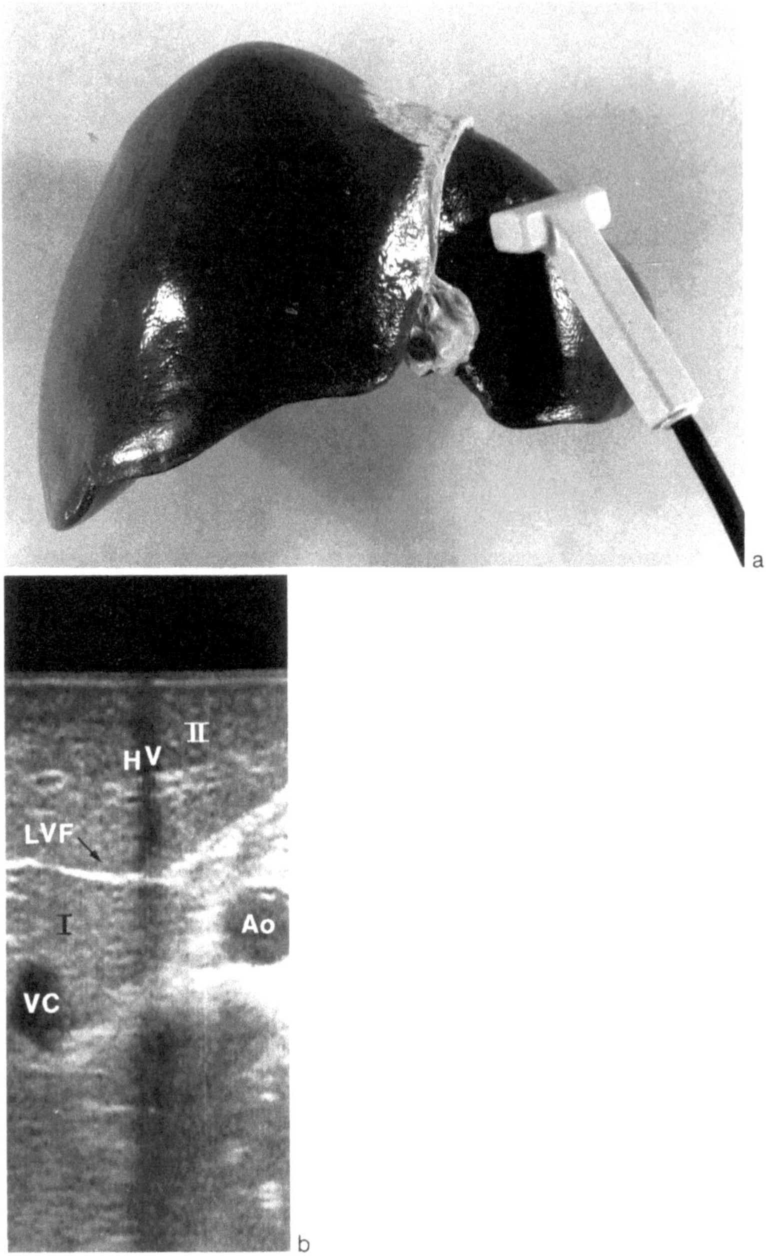

Fig. 3.33 a, b. Transverse section 5: fissure for ligamentum venosum. **a** Position of the probe. **b** Sonogram. *LVF,* fissure for ligamentum venosum; *A,* aorta; *VC,* inferior vena cava; *I,* segment I; *II,* segment II; *HV,* hepatic vein

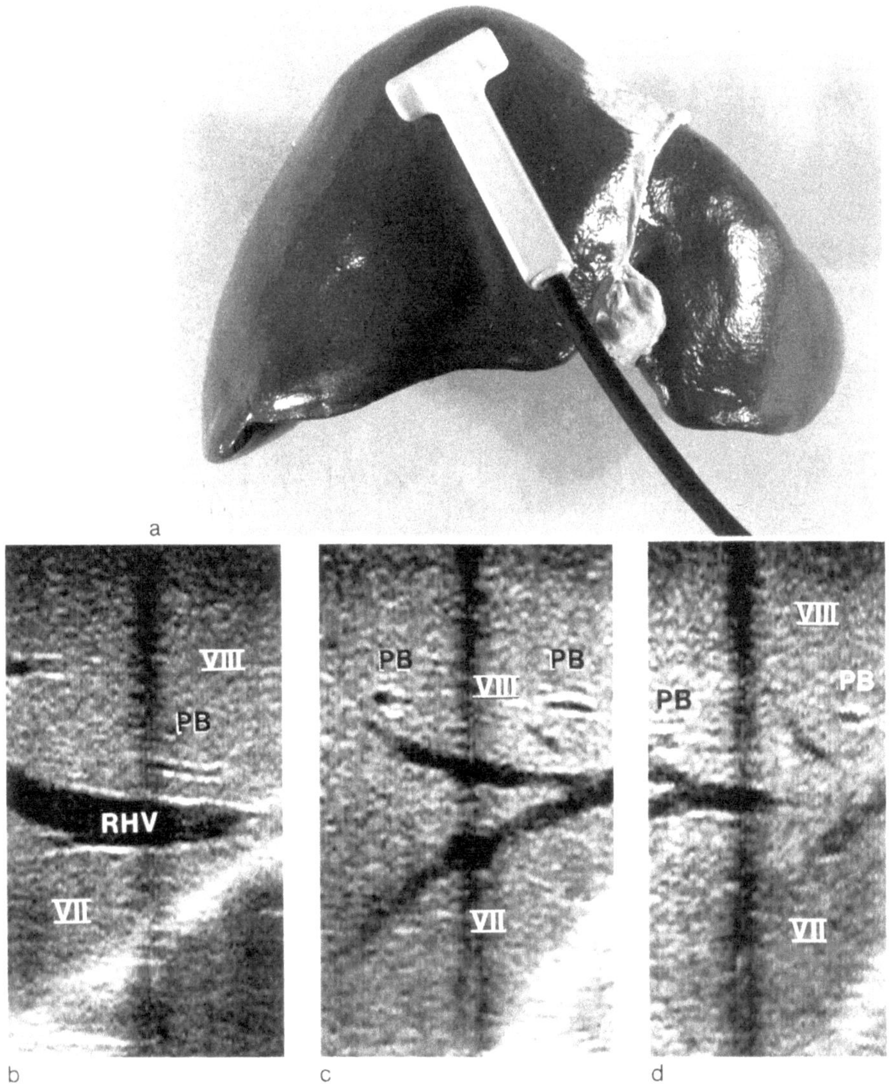

Fig. 3.34 a–d. Transverse section 6: right hepatic vein. **a** Position of the probe. This section localizes the inflow of the right hepatic vein. The ultrasound beam is directed superiorly and to the right. **b** Sonogram; *RHV*, right hepatic vein; *VII*, segment VII; *VIII*, segment VIII; *PB*, portal branch. **c, d** By slowly displacing the probe toward the anterior liver outline, while keeping the same orientation of the ultrasound beam, it is possible to follow the vein all along its course

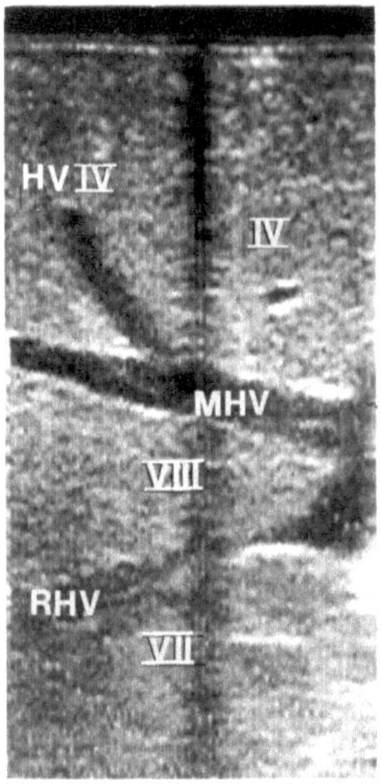

Fig. 3.35. Transverse section 7: middle hepatic vein. By recentering the probe and bringing it close to the anterior border, it is possible to discern the middle hepatic vein (*MHV*). IV, segment IV; *VIII*, segment VIII; *HV IV*, hepatic vein from segment IV

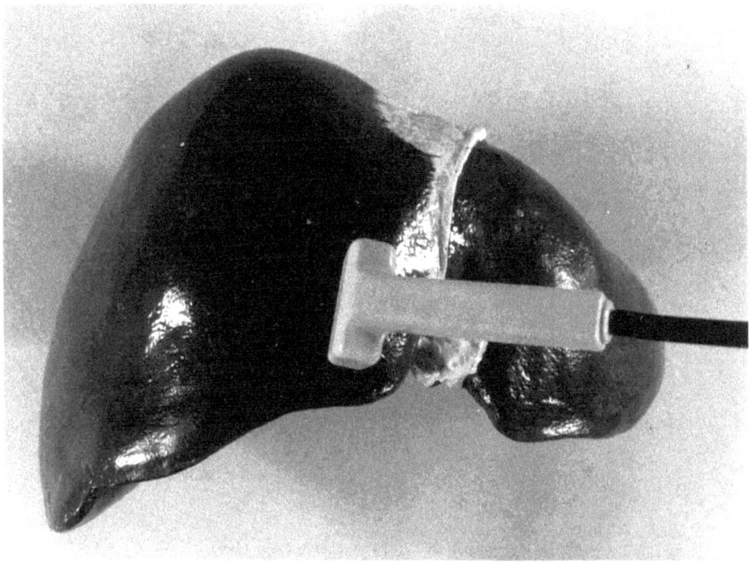

a

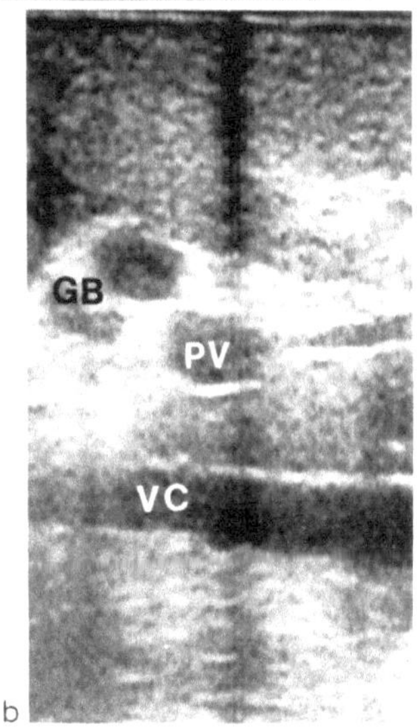

b

Fig. 3.36 a, b. Longitudinal section 1: porta hepatis. **a** Position of the probe; **b** Sonogram; *VC*, vena cava; *PV*, portal vein; *GB*, gallbladder

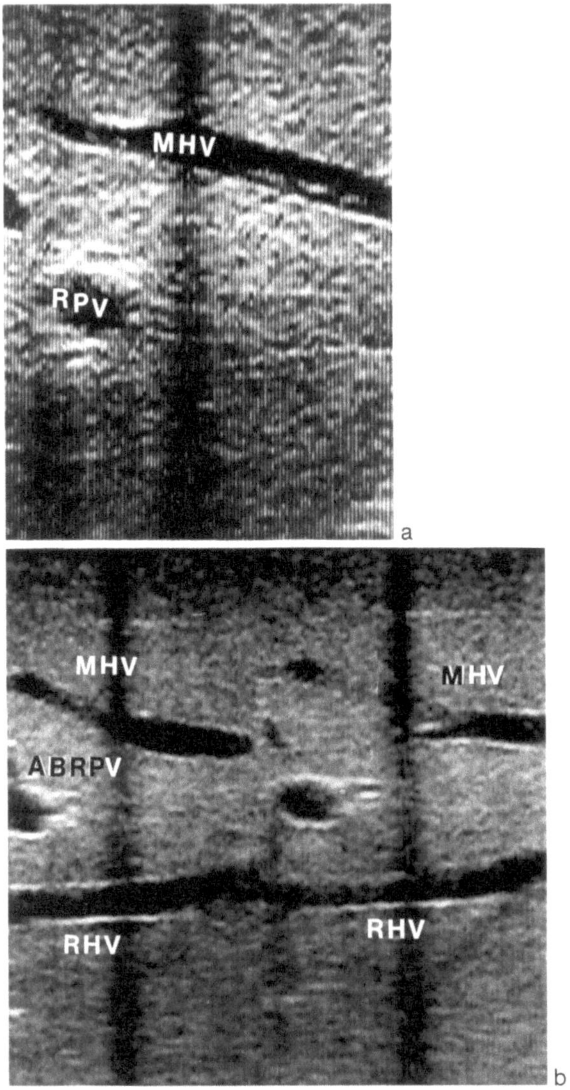

Fig. 3.37 a, b. Longitudinal section 2: middle hepatic vein. The probe is placed on a line joining the gallbladder to the left border of the inferior vena cava. **a** Sonogram; *MHV*, middle hepatic vein; *RPV*, right portal vein. **b** Variation of the preceding section, obtained by directing the ultrasound beam toward the right. *ABRPV*, anterior branch of right portal vein; *RHV*, right hepatic vein

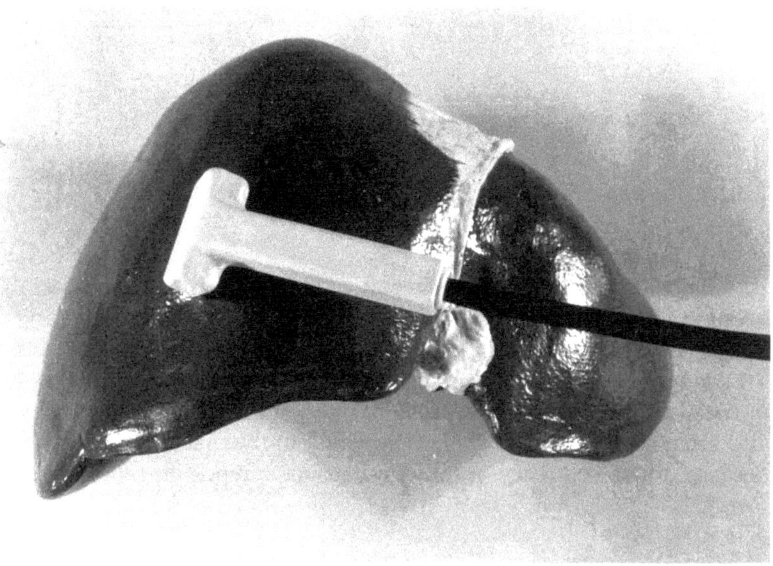

a

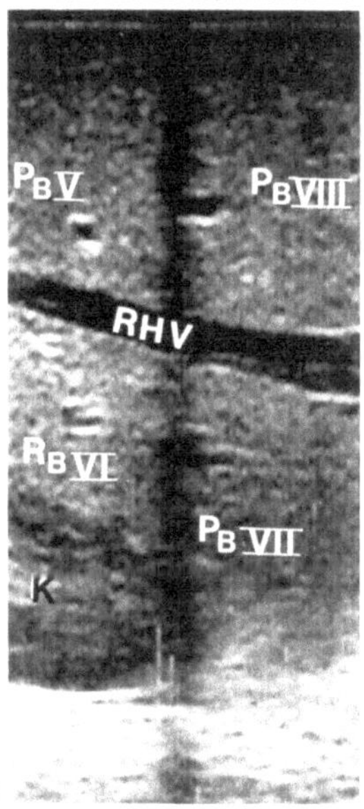

b

Fig. 3.38 a, b. Longitudinal section 3: right hepatic vein. **a** Position of the probe. **b** Sonogram; *RHV*, right hepatic vein; *PB V*, portal branch to segment V; *PB VI*, portal branch to segment VI; *PB VII*, portal branch to segment VII; *PB VIII*, portal branch to segment VIII; *K*, kidney

3.4 Synthetic Study

3.4.1 Benign Lesions

3.4.1.1 Intraoperative Ultrasound Findings

Benign Tumors

Adenomas. These are purely hepatic cell tumors that are considerably more frequent in women, promoted by the estroprogestational hormones, and complicated by the risks of hemorrhage [37]. Sonography allows recognition of the tumor, but the sonographic signs have no histological specificity. The mass may appear round or oval, and its sonographic structure may be variable. Often, it is hypoechogenic, and sometimes hyperechogenic. The center of the mass may appear heterogeneous because of the frequency of necrosis causing a hypoechogenic (even anechogenic) zone [51].

Focal Nodular Hyperplasia. This condition produces lesions that appear as rounded, mostly hypoechogenic zones. Again, they can sometimes be hyperechogenic or mixed, and can lead to a mass effect if they are voluminous [37, 47].

Hemangiomas. These are very frequent tumors, the incidence of which has been evaluated as being 2% in one autopsy series of 2400 cases [40]. In 50% of cases, hemangiomas are located in the right lobe; in 25% they are present in both lobes [14]. From the sonographic point of view, we can describe three variants [12, 13, 37, 57]:

1. A hyperechogenic image whose outline is more or less regular (Fig. 3.39).
2. A hypoechogenic image with a central septum.
3. The association of a hypoechogenic image with posterior reinforcement, suggesting a fluid content, and internal echoes.

The hyperechogenic forms appear most frequently [12]. They are generally isolated and small. Their location is quite characteristic, in that they are usually located posteriorly, in apposition to either a hepatic vein or the hepatic capsule [37].

Hepatic Abscesses

An abscess appears as a zone free of echoes that presents some echogenic zones corresponding to septa, and necrotic remnants of variable sizes. The outlines of these zones are irregular, and roughly circular. The wall of the abscess forms an irregular peripheral echo. There is not always posterior reinforcement [51, 56]. Here, ultrasonography is useful for precise localization of certain deep-seated abscesses, to exclude the presence of further lesions, and to ensure the correct arrangement of the drainage system inserted [9, 24] (Fig. 3.40).

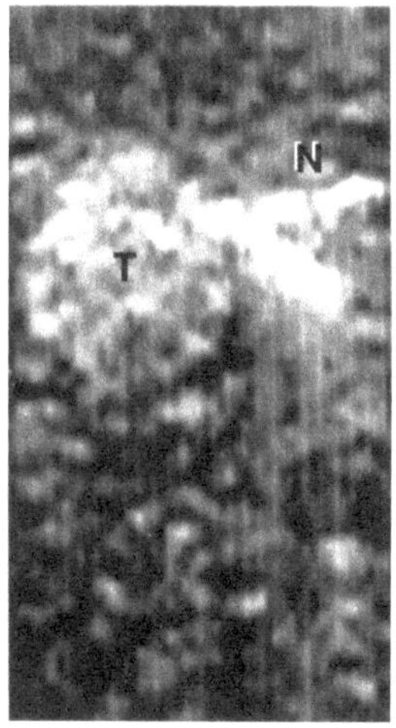

Fig. 3.39. Sonogram from a patient of 60 years with hepatic cirrhosis. During intervention for mesentericocaval deviation, ultrasonography detected a hyperechogenic image of 1 cm diameter. With regard to the history, this image suggested hepatocarcinoma on cirrhosis. The sonographically-guided puncture invalidated the diagnosis. The lesion was a hemangioma. *T*, tumor; *N*, needle

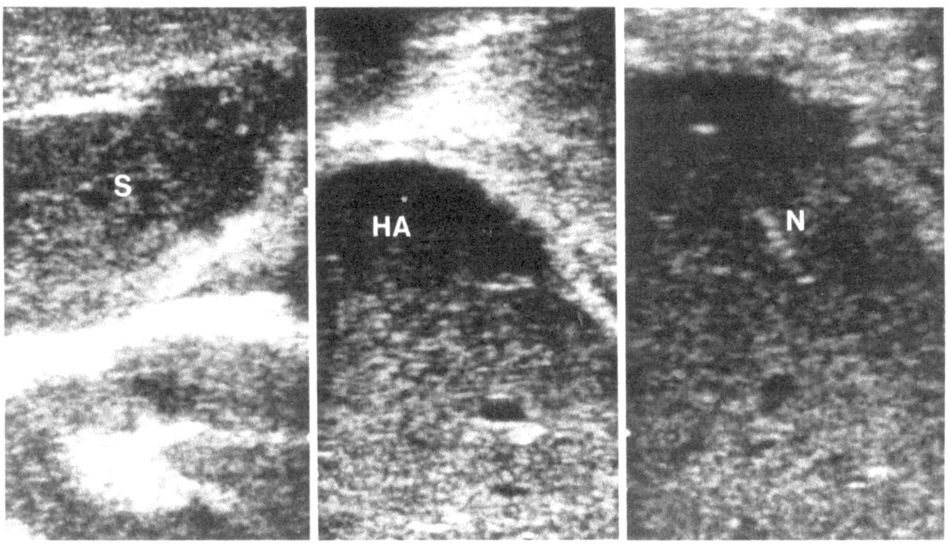

Fig. 3.40 a–c. Sonogram from a patient 25 years of age, presenting, on day 20 of hospitalization for multiple trauma, a clinical picture of acute cholecystitis. During intervention the intraoperative sonogram confirmed the diagnosis (**a**), showing a gallbladder with a thickened wall and very echogenic contents. *S*, sludge. In addition, (**b**) this examination located a hepatic abscess (*HA*) which was punctured and drained (**c**). *N*, needle

Hydatid Cyst

Solitary or multiple hydatid cysts are characterized by a well-demarcated, rounded zone of fluid nature, which is free of echo; its wall is echogenic, and is sometimes duplicated internally by a fine dense line corresponding to the germinal membrane. The existence of germinal vesicles is indicated by the presence of fine echoes located in the lower part of the cyst [23, 51, 56]. In the case of fissuration this feature disappears, resulting in a completely modified, very heterogeneous appearance [1]. In this field operative ultrasonography has no great advantage, either for diagnosis, which has usually been made prior to intervention, or for investigation regarding a possible biliary fistula, although the latter may sometimes be visualized. For this purpose, it is easier to introduce a dye into the biliary ducts or to perform cholangiography. On the other hand, ultrasonography is useful for study of the relationships of one or more cysts to neighboring structures, such as hepatic veins or the hilum, in order to avoid certain risks and adapt the surgical technique employed [9]. It can also be used to check for other small cysts that may be responsible for recurrences (Fig. 3.41).

Biliary Cysts

Although the frequency of such lesions is difficult to evaluate, Peltokaliov [43], from an autopsy series, reported an incidence of 0.16%-0.53%. In general the sonograms obtained are quite characteristic [37, 51, 56] (Fig. 3.42). They show well-demarcated, rounded or oval formations that are free of echo, and have thin, regular walls with posterior reinforcement of echoes. Their size varies from a few millimeters to several centimeters. In spite of a rather characteristic image, some could be mistaken for necrotic metastases [55, 58].

Points to keep in mind about the most frequent sonographic features of benign hepatic lesions *are that*:

1. Adenomas are usually hypoechogenic.
2. Focal nodular hyperplasia is usually hypoechogenic.
3. Hemangiomas are commonly hyperechogenic.
4. Biliary cysts are usually anechogenic.

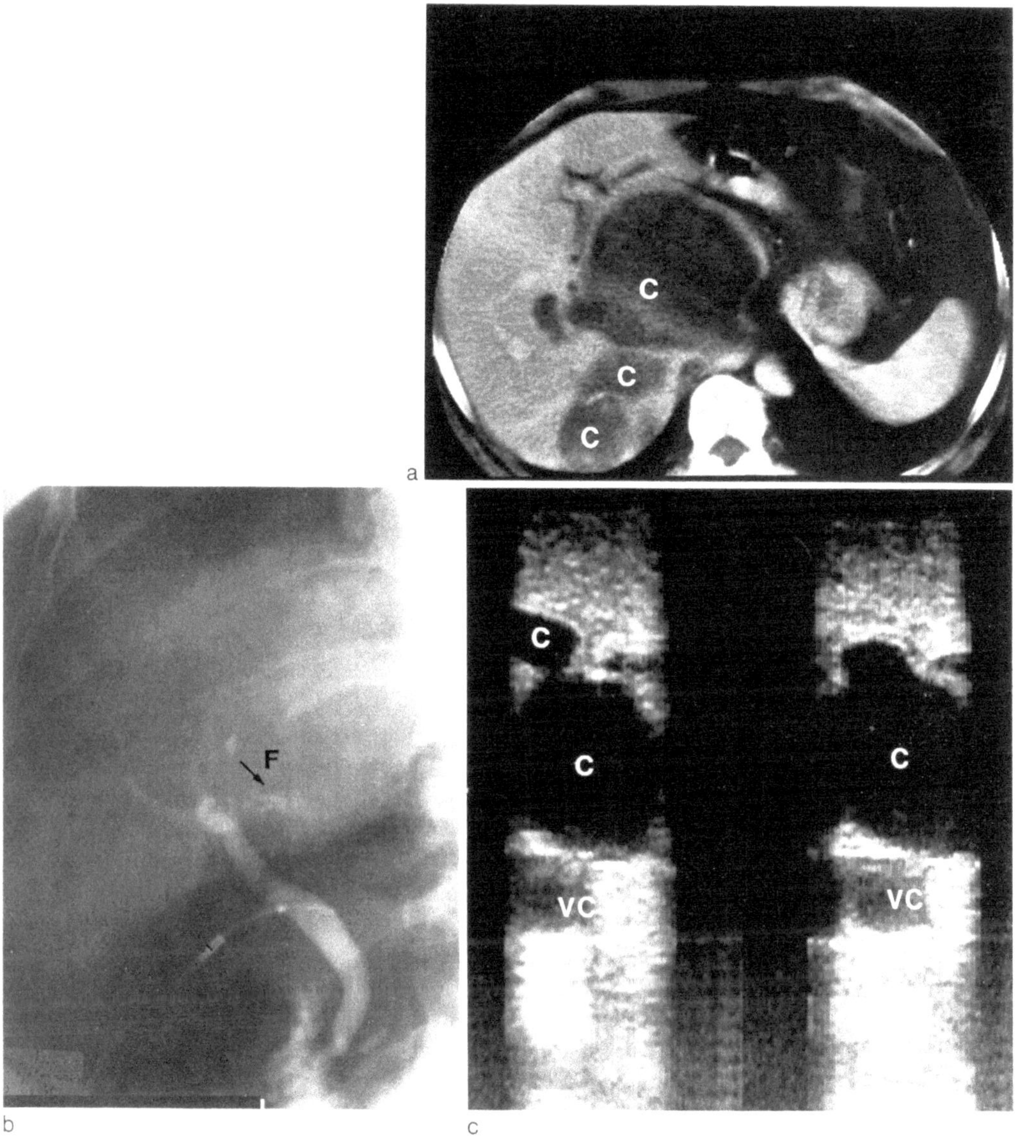

Fig. 3.41 a–c. Sonogram from a man of 57 years, hospitalized for painful hepatomegaly. The hydatic immunology was positive. CT detected a voluminous cystic formation of the liver (**a**). During intervention, cholangiography (**b**) revealed a biliary fistula (*F*). Ultrasonography (**c**) specified the intimate relations of the cyst to the vascular structures, and confirmed that all the cysts were intercommunicating; *C*, cyst; *VC*, vena cava

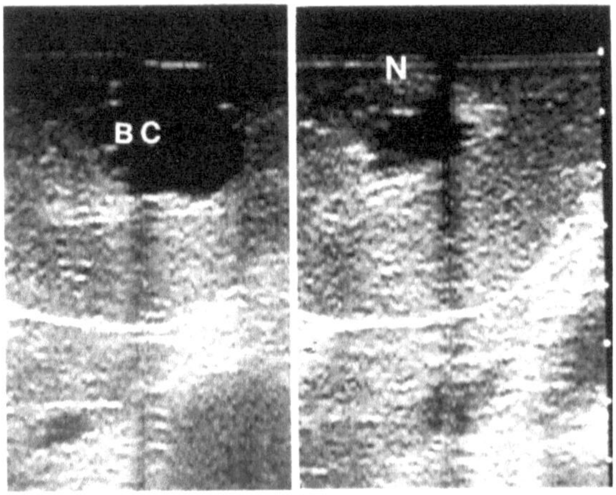

a b

Fig. 3.42 a, b. Sonogram from a patient operated upon for cancer of the colon. Intraoperative hepatic sonogram shows a rounded image free of echo with very thin walls characteristic of a biliary cyst (**a**). The puncture collapsed this formation by extracting a clear liquid whose cytologic examination proved negative (**b**); *BC*, biliary cyst; *N*, needle

3.4.1.2 Advantages and Importance of Operative Ultrasonography

The very diverse nature of the images obtained does not always allow total certitude about the exact nature of a lesion. It is well-known that under certain circumstances, e. g. gastrointestinal tumor or cirrhosis [19, 34], paraclinical investigations can detect a hepatic lesion which, although benign, may be misinterpreted as a metastasis or even as a primary malignant lesion. During surgical intervention, the same risk is present. Ultrasonography, by demonstrating the lesion and above all providing a sonographically guided biopsy, can prove that the lesion is benign. This situation may arise under several circumstances:

1. *In surgery for gastrointestinal tumors,* routine use of intraoperative sonographic examination may detect or localize a suspicious sonographic abnormality. Are we dealing with a metastasis? A sonographically guided puncture biopsy can allow us to recognize the benign nature of a lesion (see Fig. 3.42).
2. In *hepatic surgery,* as pointed out by Bismuth [11], it may be "that a surgical operation has been modified, even abandoned, when a new nodular lesion evoking a metastasis was discovered at palpation of the liver. In reality it was a benign lesion". Use of operative ultrasonography should avoid this kind of error.
3. In *surgery for portal hypertension,* sonographic exploration of the liver can sometimes detect a nodular formation that is suggestive a priori of hepatocarcinoma secondary to cirrhosis, but in fact it is a simple benign lesion (see Fig. 3.39). Ultrasound, and above all, guided puncture, permit recognition and proof of the benign nature of the lesion.

3.4.2 Hepatic Metastases

3.4.2.1 Intraoperative Ultrasound Findings

Exact knowledge of the sonographic images of lesions is less important in operative than in conventional sonography. The detection of lesions generally lies within the well-defined scope of the preoperative examinations that are performed with the aim of diagnosis. Nevertheless, description of such lesions ought to be an integral part of the operative report. This description should include the nature, size, localization and number of abnormal images. Let us briefly recall the different sonographic appearances seen [13, 56]:

- The most common abnormal feature is a rounded or oval zone that is hyperechogenic and usually heterogeneous (Fig. 3.43).
- There may be a hypoechogenic image within the hepatic parenchyma (Fig. 3.44).
- The "target" sign consists of an image formed by a hyperechogenic center surrounded by a hypoechogenic halo (Fig. 3.45).
- The "bull's eye" aspect is characterized by an echogenic corona and a center free from echoes suggestive of a liquid.
- Large metastases frequently have a hypoechogenic central necrotic zone. Certain metastases whose structure is similar to that of the parenchyma will be recognized indirectly by displacement or compression of surrounding vascular structures (Fig. 3.46). Such lesions may not be noticed even with operative ultrasonography if they do not cause a mass effect.

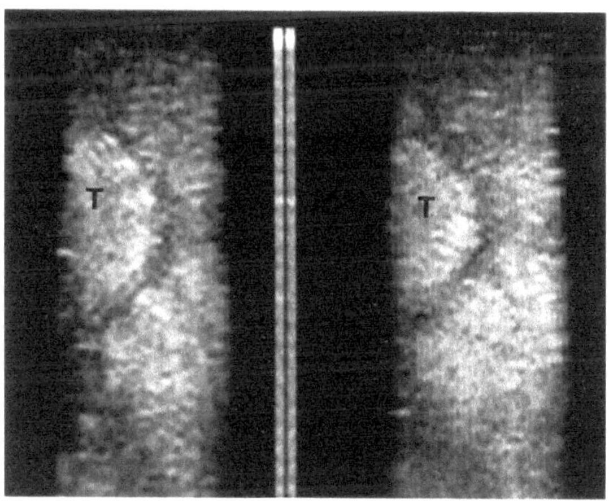

Fig. 3.43. Hyperechogenic metastasis (*T*) from cancer of the colon

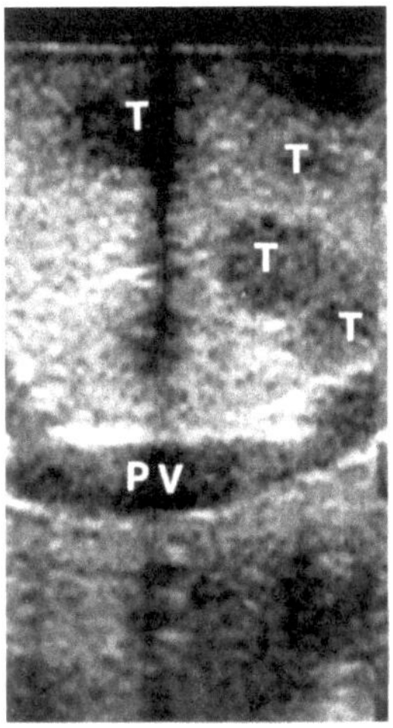

Fig. 3.44. Multiple hypoechogenic metastases (*T*) from cancer of the rectum. *PV*, portal vein

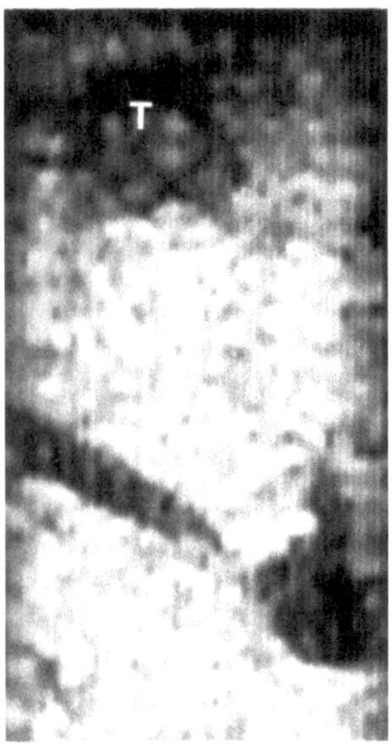

Fig. 3.45. "Target" appearance of a metastasis (*T*)

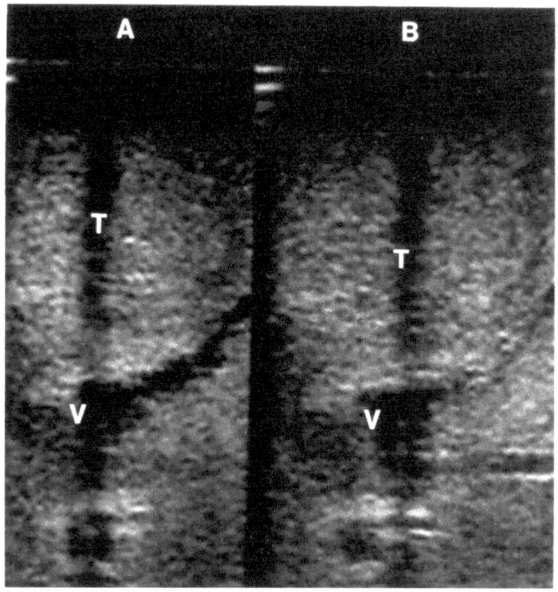

Fig. 3.46. Isoechogenic metastasis (*T*) recognized by its mass effect, displacing (*A*) and invading (*B*) the neighbouring vascular structures (*V*)

3.4.2.2 Advantages and Importance of Ultrasonography in Surgery for Gastrointestinal Tumors

Ridge and Daly [46] have evaluated the incidence of synchronous metastases of colorectal cancers as being 10%-25%. This figure was based on conventional preoperative investigations (complete biological check-up, ultrasonography, computed tomography, and/or scintigraphy) and a classical manual and visual hepatic exploration during laparotomy. In 1962, Ozarda and Pickren [41] pointed out that 11% of hepatic metastases are not demonstrated on the liver surface. Finlay et al. [20] recently reported, from repeated CT examinations, that 20% of Duke's class B and 40% of Duke's class C cancers of the colon had occult hepatic metastasis at the time of surgery. Finally, for Bengtsson et al. [7], the fact that hepatic metastasis appears during the year following curative exeresis of colorectal cancer proves that metastases were already present at the time of intervention which were undetected by preoperative investigations or intraoperative exploration. From these data, we can deduce that a certain number of metastases escape the eye and hand of the surgeon. There is of course no question of claiming to diagnose microscopic metastases by intraoperative sonography. However, due to the superiority of this examination to other investigations, in detecting nodules of less than 1 cm diameter [4, 9], we may hope to detect a certain number of "occult" metastases ([44, 45] (Fig. 3.47). Furthermore, in the case of known or visible metastasis, ultrasonography permits assessment with more certainty of the nature (by biopsy), number, and topography of the lesions [15].

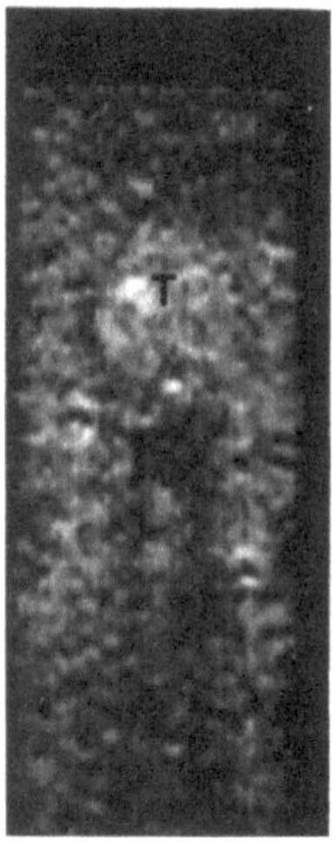

Fig. 3.47. Metastasis (*T*) of less than 1 cm diameter discovered during intervention for colonic cancer. This isolated lesion has been treated

The applications of sonographic exploration in gastrointestinal tumor surgery are numerous. In all cases, with or without metastases, this examination permits a more accurate prognosis of the primary tumor to be made. In cases of detection or confirmation of hepatic metastases, ultrasonography can reinforce or modify the therapeutic approach to the primary gastrointestinal tumor. It can help in choosing the best approach to one or more secondary lesions. Thus the surgeon will be able to remove a small metastasis during the same operative procedure. Ultrasonography can also indicate the appropriate site for an intraarterial catheter in cases of characterized diffuse or bilateral lesions. In such cases, ultrasonography can facilitate the investigation of a possible variation of the hepatic artery, without the use of preoperative angiography. In other cases, the surgeon may choose to perform a secondary surgical exeresis [27], being already aware of the precise nature of the lesion.

In cases without evidence of hepatic lesions, some authors [52] have proposed that, in colorectal cancer, it is possible to administer prophylactic intraportal chemotherapy. Intraoperative ultrasonography is an indispensable preliminary examination prior to institution of such prophylaxis.

3.4.2.3 Advantages and Application in Treatment of Hepatic Metastases

It is generally admitted that only surgery offers a chance of cure to patients with hepatic metastasis, which is usually of colorectal origin [21, 27, 46]. Unfortunately, the number of patients able to benefit from such treatment is still very limited. Several studies of metastases from colorectal cancer show that the proportion of patients for whom curative exeresis is achieved, varies between 5% and 10% [2, 3, 39, 59].

The indications for this technique, which was still risky a few years ago, are becoming more and more extended because of well-standardized techniques, the progress in intensive care, and improved understanding of hepatic regeneration [27]. The practice of operative ultrasonography in this field should improve the operative and long-term prognosis [6]. It allows the number and size of metastases to be defined. It offers the surgeon a precise map of the lesions. Furthermore, it provides very precise information about the relationships of tumoral masses to vascular elements: hepatic, portal, and vena caval (Figs. 3.48-3.50). The use of sonography in metastatic surgery has advantages on three levels [4]: for determining the indications for exeresis, for determining the type of exeresis, and for carrying out the exeresis.

Determining the Indications for Exeresis. Ultrasonography can lead to the reversal of the decision to perform exeresis because of significant dissemination or an advanced stage of tumoral extension [8]. The surgeon can then decide against therapeutic intervention or in favor of placing an intraarterial catheter for chemotherapy [4] (Fig. 3.51). Conversely, it can allow an exeresis to be performed which had appeared impossible because of the existence of disseminated lesions, if some of them are found to be benign from sonographically guided biopsies [8, 11].

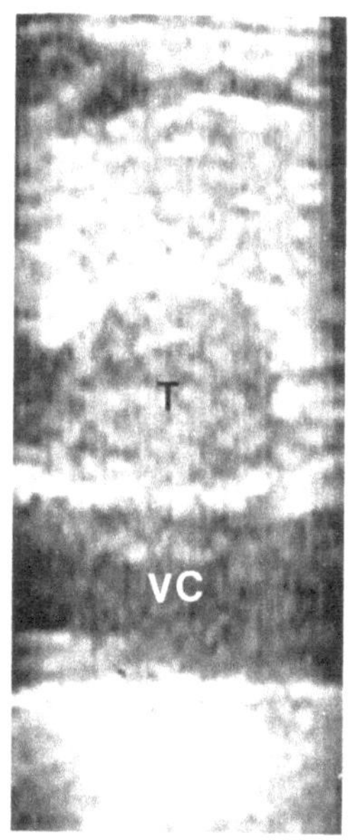

Fig. 3.48. Metastasis (*T*) from pancreatic cancer, impalpable. Note its intimate relationship to the vena cava (*VC*)

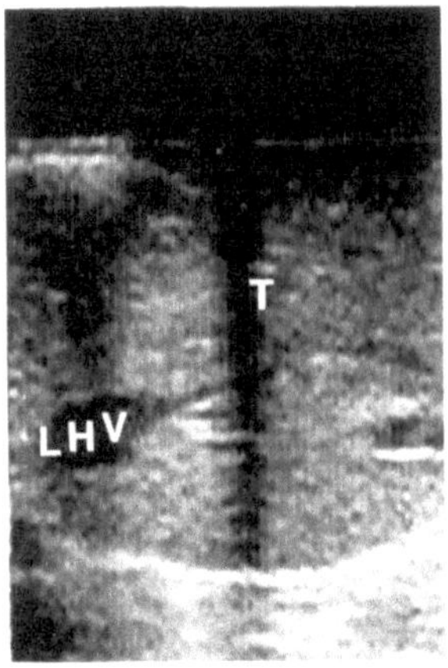

Fig. 3.49. Metastasis (*T*) from a leiomyosarcoma of the small intestine invading the left hepatic vein (*LHV*)

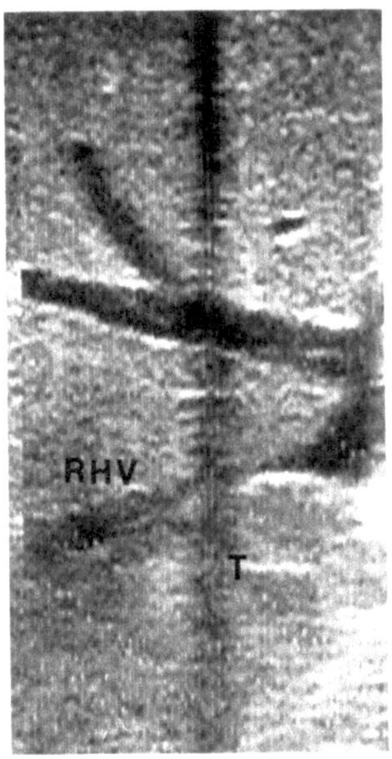

Fig. 3.50. Metastases (*T*) invading the right hepatic vein (*RHV*)

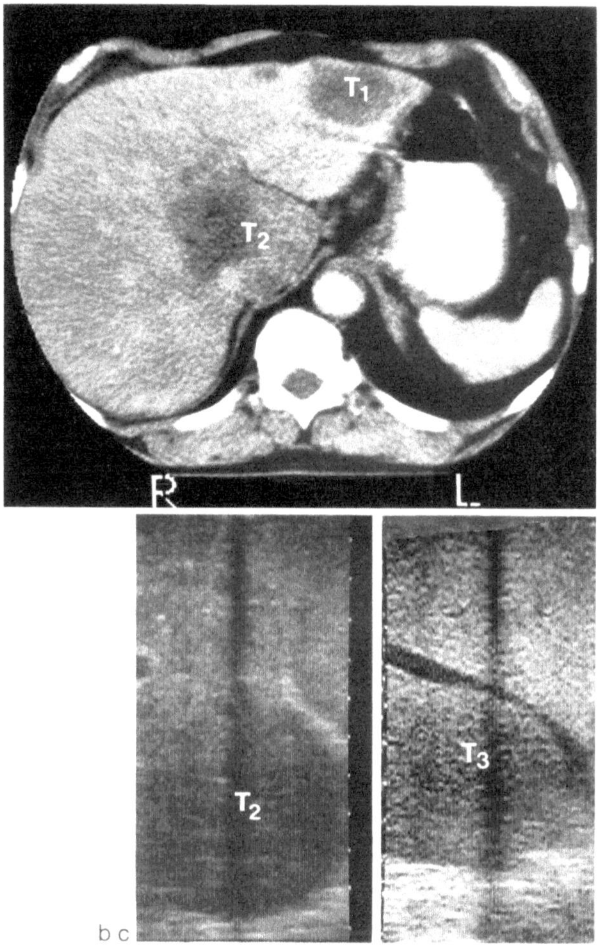

Fig. 3.51 a–c. Patient operated upon 6 months previously for colonic cancer; careful observation permits the detection of secondary hepatic lesions. The scanner (**a**) shows two predominant lesions: T_1 in segment III, and T_2 in segment I. Sonography detected the hypoechogenic lesion of segment I (T_2 in **b**) but also another site (T_3) involving and displacing the right hepatic vein (**c**)

Choice of Procedure for Exeresis. By offering the surgeon a map of the lesions, ultrasonography allows the optimal type of exeresis, considering the condition of the patient to be selected. The options can be extension of the exeresis (hepatectomy) [25], or restriction (metastasectomy [11], or segmentectomy [9]).

Performing the Exeresis. *Radical surgery* may constitute right or left hepatectomy. Ultrasonography locates the inflow of the hepatic veins, whose variations can be detected, thus eliminating the risk of gaseous embolism [4]. It identifies the precise planes of section, for instance, the main fissure, whose middle hepatic vein is a landmark and whose course can be marked on the hepatic surface with an electronic scalpel.

Otherwise, ultrasonography can discern, prior to dissection, the existence of right retrohepatic [9], median and inferior retrohepatic veins. Their importance combined with that of the middle hepatic vein can reduce the right superior hepatic vein to the role of accessory vein in 8% of cases, according to Masselot and Leborgne [35]. It is conceivable that their sonographic detection may prevent some accidents (Fig. 3.52). In addition, this examination has the advantage, upon completion of the exeresis, of verifying the integrity of the vascular elements of the remaining parenchyma [4].

Segmental surgery using ultrasonography enables noncodified and controversial metastasectomies [3, 25] to become elegant segmentectomies [10]. This is possible thanks to the identification of the portal branch irrigating the zone of interest, and to dye-injection tattooing of the exact segment to be resected. This technique, which was greatly developed in Japan [31] and worked out for hepatocarcinoma on cirrhosis, will be described later on.

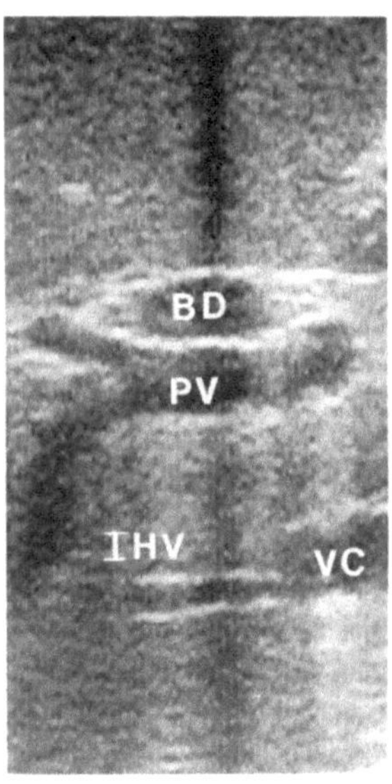

Fig. 3.52. Example of voluminous right inferior hepatic vein. *BD*, bile duct; *PV*, portal vein; *IHV*, inferior hepatic vein; *VC*, vena cava

Repeated surgery for hepatic metastases is carried out by some surgeons [8]. In this field ultrasonography acts as an indispensable anatomic guide with respect to the new hepatic architecture created by anterior resection and secondary regeneration.

Destruction of certain intrahepatic metastases by means of a laser is still an experimental technique. In the near future it will be applied clinically. Sonography will be necessary as an indispensible guide for the implementation of this technique.

3.4.3 Hepatocarcinoma on Cirrhosis

The first problem that we hepatic surgeons encountered was the invisible and impalpable tumor. Of patients with small hepatocellular carcinomas under 5 cm in diameter and cirrhosis of the liver, 60% had a nonvisible, impalpable tumor. This point makes it quite clear that hepatic surgeons need to recognize the necessity for intraoperative sonography. Apart from this, new small nodules which have not been detected by preoperative examination can be detected by intraoperative sonography. These include not only nodules of hepatocellular carcinoma but also benign lesions such as regenerative nodules, hyperplastic nodules, and hemangiomas. These nodules cannot be distinguished on the basis of sonographic patterns or aspiration cytology, but can be diagnosed by needle biopsy or enucleation. The sensitivity of intraoperative sonography in detecting small nodules in the liver is twice that of preoperative examination.

Tumor thrombus is a characteristic extension of hepatocellular carcinoma. Operative sonography is three times as sensitive in detecting tumor thrombus as preoperative examination is (Fig. 3.53). Sonography is the only diagnostic modality that can simultaneously demonstrate the portal venous branches and the hepatic veins. With its use, visualization of the three-dimensional nature of the tumor and the hepatic vessels becomes possible. This is much easier with intraoperative sonography than with preoperative sonography. If during transection of the liver, unknown vessels are exposed on the cut surface of the liver, they can be identified sonographically. The plane transecting the liver is demonstrated as an echogenic line (Fig. 3.54). Therefore the plane of transection can be suitably oriented. Moreover, intraoperative sonography has fostered two new operative procedures for hepatectomy. One is systematic subsegmentectomy [30, 31] and the other is hepatectomy preserving the right inferior hepatic vein [32].

Systematic subsegmentectomy is indicated for patients with a small hepatocellular carcinoma and impaired hepatic function due to cirrhosis. The operative procedure comprises intraoperative sonography to establish the distribution of vessels with respect to the tumor, sonographically guided puncture of the portal venous branch to identify the portal area containing the tumor, and tattooing to indicate the ligation point of the vessels (Fig. 3.55). This operation is conducted for total resection of a small portal area containing tumor, because cancer cells of hepatocellular carcinoma are spread via the portal venous branches. Systematic subsegmentectomy is generally accepted among Japanese hepatic surgeons as a standard radical operation for small hepatocellular carcinoma associated with cirrhosis [53].

If a right inferior hepatic vein is present (20%-24% of cases) [32], partial hepatectomies protecting the posteroinferior right region can also be carried out. These interventions allow partial hepatectomies in patients with altered hepatic functions. Intraoperative sonography becomes here a necessity.

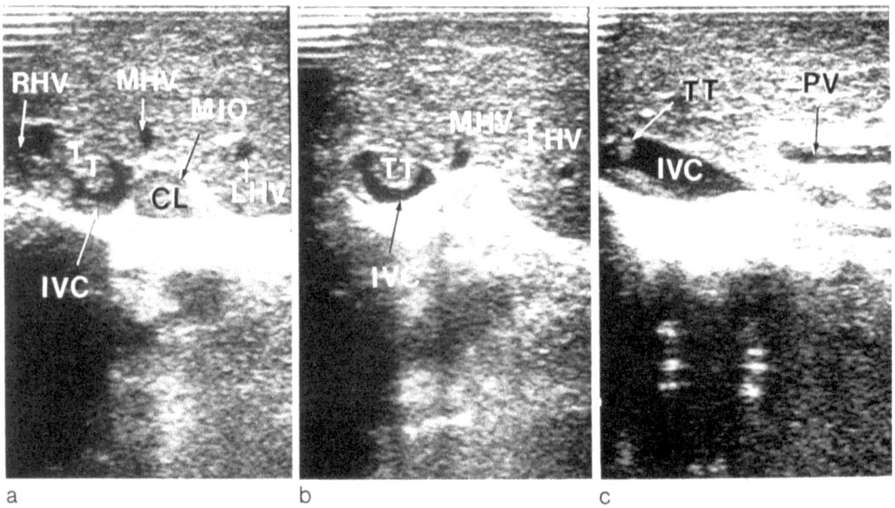

Fig. 3.53 a–c. Intraoperative sonograms of tumor thrombus. This patient has a hepatocellular carcinoma 5 cm in diameter in the right posterosuperior area (segment VII). Preoperative examinations such as sonography, computed tomography, hepatic arteriography and hepatic venography had not detected tumor thrombus. However, intraoperative sonography demonstrated a tumor thrombus in the right hepatic vein and the inferior vena cava. **a** Transverse sonogram of the right hepatic vein and the inferior vena cava. At the confluence of the right hepatic vein (*RHV*) and the inferior vena cava (*IVC*), tumor thrombus (*TT*) is seen. *MHV*, middle hepatic vein; *LHV*, left hepatic vein; *MiO*, minor (lesser) omentum; *CL*, caudate lobe. **b** Transverse sonogram slightly cranial to **a.** Round and oval tumor thrombus is seen in the inferior vena cava. **c** Longitudinal sonogram of the inferior vena cava. At the cranial end of the inferior vena cava, tumor thrombus is demonstrated. *PV*, portal vein

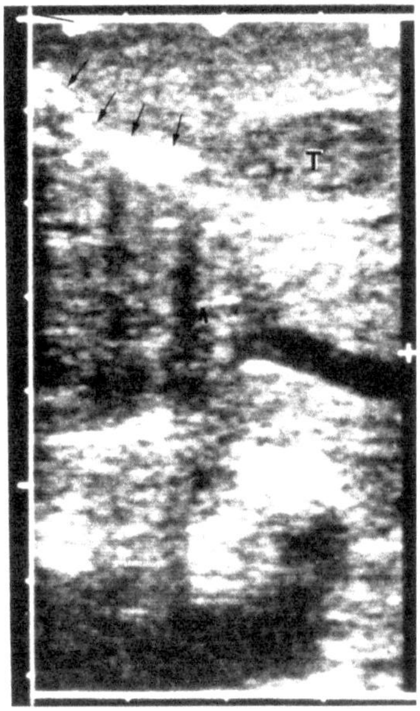

Fig. 3.54. Intraoperative sonogram of the transecting plane of the liver parenchyma. During division of the parenchyma, after the cut surfaces of the liver had been replaced in the natural position, the diaphragmatic surface of the liver was scanned. The transecting plane (*arrows*) is delineated as an echogenic line. Interrelations between the boundary of the liver and the tumor (*T*) indicate the direction of hepatic transection

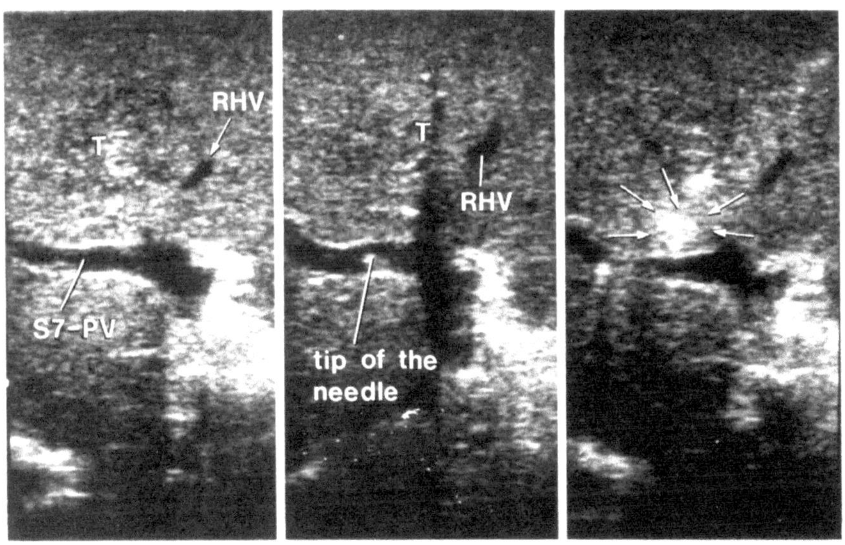

Fig. 3.55 a–c. Puncture of the portal vein and tattooing. **a** Operative sonogram of the tumor (*T*), the right hepatic vein (*RHV*) and the portal venous branch to the posterosuperior area segment VII (*S 7-PV*). **b** The portal venous branch to the posterosuperior area has been punctured, and tip of the needle is clearly seen in the portal vein. **c** Tattooing of the liver parenchyma. Injected blue dye (*arrows*) is recognized as an echogenic mass

References

1. Abdeselem K, Hassine N, Gharbi HA (1982) Complications du kyste hydatique du foie. Diagnostic échographique. Med Chir Dig 11: 189-191
2. Adson MA (1983) Hepatic metastases in perspective. AJR 140: 695-700
3. Adson MA, Van Heerden JA (1980) Major hepatic resections for metastatic colorectal cancer. Ann Surg 191: 576-583
4. Alexandre JH, Hernigou A, Bouillot JL, Plainfosse MCH, Billebaud TH (1985) Apport de l'échographie per-opératoire dans les métastases hépatiques. Ann Gastroenterol Hepatol 21: 27-29
5. Agossou-Voyeme AK (1982) La segmentation hépatique en tomodensitométrie. Mémoire du Laboratoire d'Anatomie des St Pères I, Paris, France
6. Belghiti J, Menu Y, Nayuh H, Fekete F (1984) Apport de l'échotomographie per-opératoire dans la chirurgie des tumeurs du foie. Presse Med 13-30: 1839-1841
7. Bengtsson G, Carlsson G, Hafström L, Johnsson PE (1981) Natural history of patients with untreated liver metastases from colorectal cancer. Am J Surg 141: 586-589
8. Bismuth H, Castaing D (1984) Traitement chirurgical des métastases hépatiques. Med Chir Dig 13: 11-12
9. Bismuth H, Castaing D (1985) Echographie per-opératoire du foie et des voies biliaires. Ed Flammarion Médecine Sciences, Paris, France
10. Bismuth H, Houssin D, Castaing D (1982) Major and minor segmentectomies in liver surgery. World J Surg 6: 10-24
11. Bismuth H, Castaing D, Kunstlinger F (1984) L'échographie per-opératoire en chirurgie hépato-biliaire. Presse Med 13: 1819-1822
12. Brun PH, Belloir A, Costaz R, Rohmer P, Weill F (1983) Etude comparative échographique et scannographique d'une série de 19 angiomes hépatiques. J Radiol 64: 15-19
13. Bruneton JN, Dageville X, Fenart D, Caramella E, Rouy P, Ocelli JP, Bourry J (1982) Les masses hépatiques en échographie. A propos de 400 cas. J Radiol 63: 181-187
14. Buffet C, Fritsch J, Etienne JP (1982) Hémangiomes géants du foie chez l'adulte, à propos de 3 cas. Gastroenterol Clin Biol 6: 531-538
15. Castaing D, Bismuth H (1984) Intérêt échographique per-opératoire dans la chirurgie des tumeurs secondaires du foie. Med Chir Dig 13, 3: 8-9
16. Couinaud C (1957) Le foie, études anatomiques et chirurgicales. Masson, Paris, France
17. Duvauferrier R, Duvauferrier-Pellenc MC, Simon J, Duval JM (1980) Anatomie échographique du foie (systématisation, variantes et images pièges), Ultrasons 1: 113-119
18. Flament JB, Delatre JE, Palot JP, Ducasse A (1985) Rappel anatomoradiologique. Ann Gastroenterol Hépatol 21: 3-11
19. Fletcher MS, Everett WG, Hunter JO (1980) Benign liver nodules presenting as apparent hepatic metastases, a report of 5 cases. Br J Surg 67: 403-405
20. Finlay IG, Meek DR, Gray HW, Duncan JG, McArdle CS (1982) Incidence and detection of occult hepatic metastases in colorectal carcinoma. Br Med J 284: 803-805
21. Foster JH, Lundy J (1981) Liver metastases. Curr Probl Surg 18: 158-202
22. Gest H, Lemaitre G (1982) Les vaisseaux intra-hépatiques normaux. Considération sur leur image échographique. J Radiol 63: 527-533
23. Gharbi HA, Hassine W, Brauner M, Dupuch K (1981) Ultrasound examination of the hydatic liver. Radiology 139: 459-463
24. Glen PM, Noseworthy J, Babcock DS (1984) Use of intra-operative ultrasonography of localized hepatic abscess. Arch Surg, Vol 119: 347-348
25. Guntz H, Cronier P, Lorimier G, Dabadie V (1985) Les possibilités chirurgicales dans le traitement des métastases hépatiques. Ann Gastroenterol 21: 67-72
26. Huguet C, Nordlinger B, Cunci O, Parc R (1985) Résection chirurgicale des métastases hépatiques des cancers du côlon et du rectum. A propos de 49 cas. Ann Gastroenterol Hepatol 21: 73-74
27. Joyeux H, Solassol C (1983) Possibilités chirurgicales actuelles dans le traitement des métastases hépatiques des adénocarcinomes colo-rectaux. Gastroenterol Clin Biol 7: 237-239
28. Kane RA (1981) Sonographic anatomy of the liver. Semin Ultrasound 2: 190-197

29. Lortat-Jacob JL, Robert HG, Henry C (1952) Un cas d'hépatectomie droite réglée. Mem Acad Chir 78: 244-251
30. Makuuchi M, Hasegawa H, Yamasaki S (1981) Intra-operative ultrasonic examination for hepatectomy. Jpn J Clin Oncol 11: 367-390
31. Makuuchi M, Hasegawa H, Yamazaki S (1985) Ultrasonically guided subsegmentectomy. Surg Gynecol Obstet 161: 346-350
32. Makuuchi M et al (1987) Inferior right hepatic vein preserving hepatectomies. Surg Gynecol Obstet 164: 69-72
33. Marks WM, Filly RA, Callen PW (1979) Ultrasonic anatomy of the liver: a review with new applications. J Clin Ultrasound 7: 137-146
34. Martelli H, Tubiana JM (1982) Découverte de lésions bénignes du foie lors du dépistage de métastases hépatiques. Nouv Presse Med 11: 2833-2836
35. Masselot R, Leborgne J (1985) Etude anatomique des veines sus-hépatiques. Anat Clin 1: 109-125
36. Melliere D (1966) Topographie artérielle et chirurgie pancréatique. Thèse médecine, Paris, France
37. Menu Y, Scherrer A, Grenier P, Nahum H (1984) L'échographie des tumeurs bénignes du foie chez l'adulte. Rev Praticien 34: 351-355
38. Michels NA (1955) Blood supply and anatomy of the upper abdominal organs, Lippincott & Co, Philadelphia, USA pp 152-154, 256-259, 374-375
39. Nordlinger A, De Sena G, Szawlowski A, Orea Martinez JG, Parc R, Malafosse M, Huguet C (1983) Résection chirurgicale des métastases hépatiques des cancers du côlon et du rectum. Gastroenterol Clin Biol 7: 240-243
40. Ochsner JL, Halpert B (1958) Cavernous hemangioma of the liver. Surgery 43: 557
41. Ozarda A, Pickren J (1962) The topographic distribution of the liver metastases, its relation to surgical and isotopic diagnosis. J Nucl Med 3: 149-152
42. Parulekar SG (1979) Ligaments and fissures of the liver: sonographic anatomy. Radiology 130: 409-411
43. Peltokallio V (1970) Non parasitic cysts of the liver. A clinical study of 117 cases. Ann Chir Gynaecol Fenn [Suppl] 59: 174-1+
44. Plainfosse MC, Merran S (1983) Work in progress: intra-operative abdominal ultrasound. Radiology 147: 829-832
45. Plainfosse MC, Hernigou A, Merran S (1983) L'échographie per-opératoire en chirurgie digestive. Med Chir Dig 12: 493-496
46. Ridge JA, Daly JM (1985) Treatment of colorectal hepatic metastases. Surg Gynecol Obstet 161: 597-607
47. Roger JV, Mack LA, Freeny PC et al (1981) Hepatic focal nodular hyperplasia. Angiography, CT, sonography and scintigraphy. Am J Radiol 137: 983-990
48. Senecail B, Memanteau B, Quereux P (1980) Hepatic tomo-anatomy, introduction to the echo-anatomy of the normal liver. Anat Clin 2: 181-190
49. Senegas J, Rigaud A (1969) Etude de l'artériographie du foie humain et de ses variations en fonction de la forme et de l'orientation de ce viscère. Bull Assoc Anat 143: 1535-1544
50. Sexton CC, Zehan RK (1983) Correlation of computed tomography, sonography and gross anatomy of the liver. AJR 141: 711-718
51. Taboury J (1980) Guide pratique d'échographie abdominale. Ed Masson, Paris, France, Chap 4: 23-43
52. Taylor I, West C, Rowling J (1982) Can colorectal liver metastases be prevented? In: Gerar A (ed) Progress and perspectives in the treatment of gastro-intestinal tumors. Pergamon, Oxford, pp 89-92
53. Tobe T (1984) Hepatectomy in patients with cirrhotic liver: clinical and basic observations. In: Nyhus LM (ed) Surgery Annual. Appleton-Century-Crofts, Norwalk, Connecticut, pp 177-202
54. Ton That Tung (1979) Les résections majeures et mineures du foie. Ed Masson, Paris, France, 1-36
55. Weaver RH, Goldstein HM, Green B, Perkins C (1978) Grey scale ultrasonographic evaluation of hepatic cystic disease. AJR 130: 849-852
56. Weill FS (1981) Ultrasonographie en pathologie digestive. Ed Vigot Frères, Paris, France

57. Weiner SN, Parulekar SG (1979) Scintigraphy and sonography of hepatic hemangioma. Radiology 132: 149-151
58. Wooten WB, Green B, Goldstein HM (1978) Ultrasonography of necrotic hepatic metastases. Radiology 128: 447-450
59. Zerbib M, Place S, Bonnichon P, Pinto P, Delaitre B, Chapuis Y (1985) Evaluation du nombre de métastases susceptibles de faire l'objet d'un traitement chirurgical de métastases hépatiques. A partir d'une série de 180 cancers colorectaux. Ann Gastroenterol Hepatol 21: 63-65

4 Ultrasonography of the Biliary Tract

B. Deixonne, F.-M. Lopez, M. Makuuchi, A. Pissas

4.1 Introduction

Apart from its role in surgery, in current medical practice sonography enables us to carry out a very satisfactory exploration of the biliary tract. Furthermore, in biliary pathology, it is emerging as a good examination among other methods, assuming first place in investigative imaging. On the basis of this, one is tempted to think that intraoperative sonography should play the same primary role. Experience proves this to be very difficult. During biliary intervention, it is easy to perform cholangiography, which does not take much longer than sonography. Classical radiomanometry is still sometimes used. Otherwise, if necessary, the surgeon can complete the exploration of the common bile duct by choledochoscopy. For a long time, surgeons have been well acquainted with these three techniques, which on the whole are satisfying. Thus, in intraoperative biliary tract exploration, sonography appears to be a new method providing only the same information as the existing widely disseminated methods. We shall see that this assumption should be qualified.

4.2 Surgical Anatomy of the Biliary Tract

There are two extrahepatic biliary ducts: the common bile duct and the accessory biliary apparatus.

4.2.1 The Common Bile Duct

The intrahepatic ducts join together at the hilum of the liver (superior biliary confluence) to form the common hepatic duct (ductus hepaticus communis). The latter becomes the common bile duct (ductus choledochus) after receiving the cystic duct. The common bile duct opens into the medial side of the second part of the duodenum (Fig. 4.1). The common hepatic duct usually commences at the hilum of the liver. It is formed by the junction of both hepatic ducts, the right and the left, anterior to the right branch of the portal vein, posteriorly, superiorly, and to

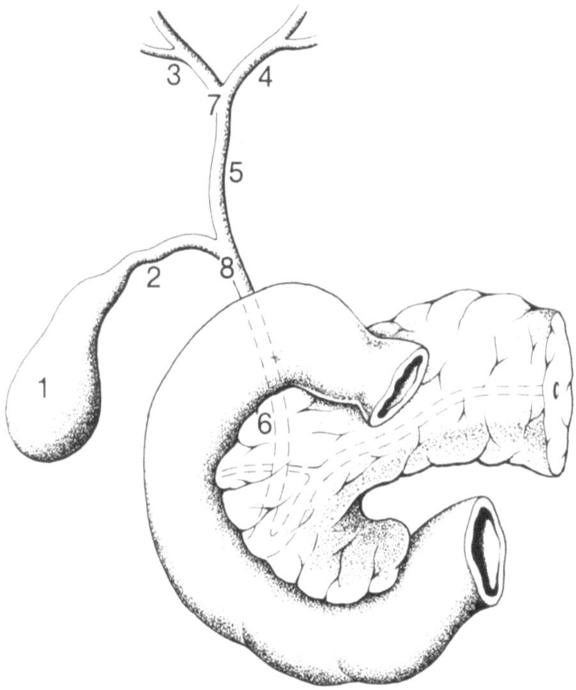

Fig. 4.1. Biliary tract; *1, 2,* accessory biliary apparatus: *1,* gallbladder; *2,* cystic duct; *3–8,* principal biliary apparatus: *3,* right hepatic duct; *4,* left hepatic duct; *5,* common bile duct; *6,* retropancreatic portion of common bile duct; *7,* superior biliary convergence; *8,* inferior biliary convergence

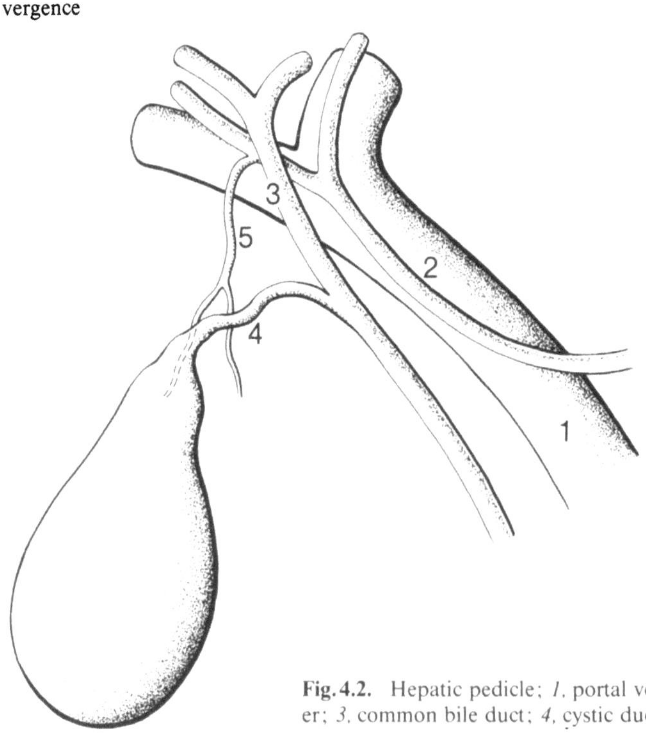

Fig. 4.2. Hepatic pedicle; *1,* portal vein; *2,* hepatic artery proper; *3,* common bile duct; *4,* cystic duct; *5,* cystic artery

the right of the division of the hepatic artery. This classical arrangement has a great number of variations involving the more or less early confluence of the right and left sectorial ducts. The superior biliary confluence is situated in direct apposition to the superior aspect of the hilar plate, without any vascular interposition; it is possible to approach it directly by freeing the hilar plate and opening the main fissure.

The common bile duct is situated in the free edge of the lesser omentum anterior to the right side of the portal trunk (Fig. 4.2). It moves away from the lower part of the pedicle, describing an interportocholedochal triangle. The hepatic artery ascends on the left side of the portal vein and is divided into a right and left branch superior to the initial part of the common bile duct. To reach the liver, the right branch crosses the common bile duct, usually posteriorly, but sometimes anteriorly. The cystic artery, varying in length, arises from the hepatic artery, and usually crosses the anterior face of the common bile duct.

The gallbladder and the cystic duct are related to the right side of the common bile duct. The hepatic pedicle, completed by the nerves and lymphatic vessels, is related posteriorly to the epiploic foramen (of Winslow), forming its anterior limits. It is separated by the latter from the inferior vena cava, located posterior to the foramen. Anteriorly and inferiorly, the lower part of the pedicle is covered by the posterior surface of the first part of the duodenum. The peritoneum is reflected from the posterior side of the latter. To expose the inferior segment of the pedicle, the intestinal segment has to be pulled down. Also, the liver covering this entire region has to be lifted. At the base of the hepatic pedicle, the biliary duct is associated with the fixed region of the first part of the duodenum. The common bile duct then slopes to the posterior aspect of the pancreas where it digs out a deep groove, even forming a tunnel. The common bile duct is included in the duodenopancreatic recess and cannot be approached other than by Kocher's maneuver (retroduodenopancreatic detachment).

At the junction of the posterior and interior aspects of the second part of the duodenum in its median part, 3-4 cm from the pylorus, the common bile duct pierces the duodenal wall obliquely, adherent for 1 cm to the main pancreatic duct (of Wirsung). The site of this implantation is in fact very variable (from the genu superius to the duodenojejunal angle). The termination of the biliary and pancreatic ducts is provided with a sphincter: the sphincter of Oddi, which impedes reflux. The sphincter is composed of three parts (Fig. 4.3): a common sphincter which surrounds both ducts before they form or do not form a common duct or hepatopancreatic ampulla (of Vater); a separate sphincter for the common bile duct itself; a separate sphincter for the main pancreatic duct (of Wirsung). This sphincterial block is lodged in an opening in the internal wall of the muscular layer of the duodenum: the duodenal window.

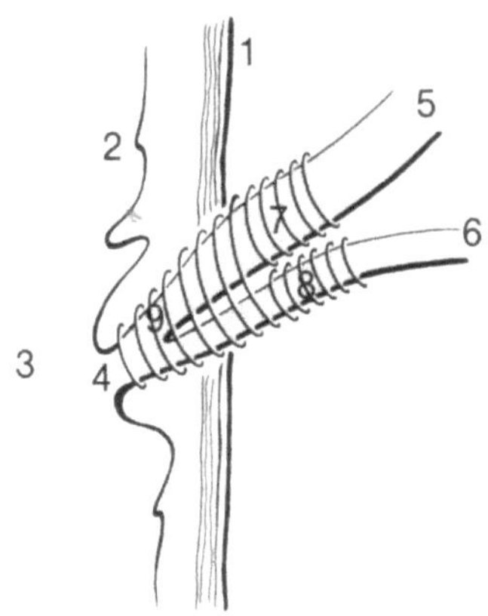

Fig. 4.3. The sphincter of Oddi; *1*, duodenal muscularis; *2*, duodenal mucosal spur; *3*, major duodenal papilla; *4*, ampulla of Vater; *5*, common bile duct; *6*, principal pancreatic duct; *7*, sphincter of common bile duct; *8*, sphincter of principal pancreatic duct; *9*, common sphincter or sphincter of Oddi

4.2.2 The Accessory Biliary Apparatus

This is composed of the gallbladder and the cystic duct (see Fig. 4.1). The gallbladder is pear-shaped, 8–10 cm long and 3–4 cm wide and situated in the variably deep cystic fossa. The rounded fundus is located at the level of the cystic notch on the liver's anterior border. The body presents a superior surface adherent to the liver and a free inferior surface covered with peritoneum. The gallbladder is oriented obliquely, sloping superiorly, posteriorly and to the left. It is constricted posteriorly, to form the 2-cm-long neck which is oriented obliquely, anteriorly, and to the right. The neck forms an acute angle, open anteriorly, with the body. It is located inferior to and to the left of the posterior extremity of the body and is dilated in its median part.

The cystic duct is 3–4 cm long. It forms an acute angle, open posteriorly, with the neck. It is oriented to the left and posteroinferiorly, apposed to the right side of the common bile duct. It usually ends slightly superior to the duodenum. The cystic duct sometimes has a spiral mucosal valve (Heister's valve). Its caliber is approximately 3 mm. Its junction with the common bile duct forms the inferior biliary confluence. Variations in its arrangement are very frequent. Notably, the opening of the cystic duct may occur at different levels.

The superior surface of the gallbladder is in contact with the thickened region of the vasculobiliary envelope covering the cystic fossa (vesicular sheath). This lamina contains the vessels of the gallbladder. The veins penetrate the lamina and enter the hepatic parenchyma. Some biliary ductules drain directly through the superior surface of the gallbladder. The inferior surface is free, and is covered with peritoneum (Fig. 4.4). It lies on the right part of the transverse colon, anteriorly, and the supramesocolic duodenum, posteriorly. The fundus of the gallbladder extends beyond the anterior border of the liver, and is directly related to the anterior abdominal wall. Sometimes the gallbladder is connected to the liver by a layer of

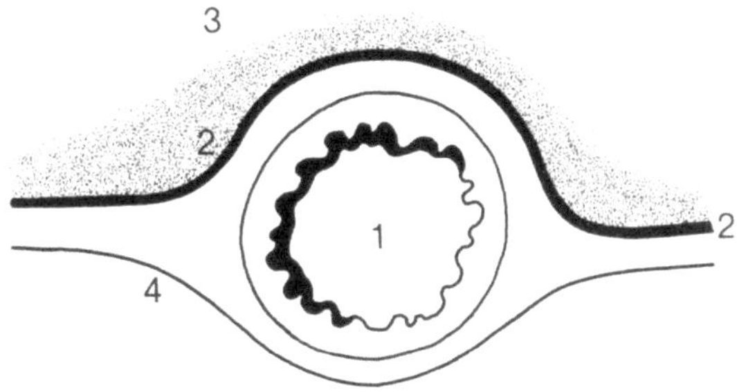

Fig. 4.4. The gallbladder bed; *1*, gallbladder; *2*, vesicular plate; *3*, liver; *4*, peritoneum

peritoneum containing vessels (the mesocyst). The neck is directly related to the right part of the porta hepatis, and consequently to the right side of the hepatic pedicle.

The cystic duct, with its usual variability, is related laterally to the common bile duct for several centimeters. Dissection allows the separation of the elements and defines the "triangle of cholecystectomy" (the left edge represents the cystic duct; the right edge, the common hepatic duct; and the superior edge, the liver), in proximity to which we find the cystic vessels, and occasionally the right branch of the hepatic artery, or the right sectorial or segmental hepatic duct.

4.3 Technical Exploration and Ultrasound Findings

The surgical approach must allow good access to the extrahepatic biliary ducts, which have to be well exposed. Apart from some exceptions, in biliary surgery we use a right subcostal approach from the median line to the angle of the ninth right rib. In order to obtain a good exposure of the subhepatic region, we section both the ligamentum teres and the cystico-duodenocolic ligament. In this way the gallbladder and the hepatic pedicle are accessible to sonographic exploration. We further recommend Kocher's maneuver for 2 or 3 cm, which permits the probe to be placed at different angles in relation to the common bile duct in its retropancreatic course. This may be useful in some difficult cases with small calculi at this level.

What kind of apparatus should be used? For extrahepatic biliary ducts one can use a linear or a sectorial probe. The cumbersomeness of the latter does not matter very much. It allows distinct visualization of all the extrahepatic biliary ducts, and by means of a hilar approach the last few centimeters of the right and left hepatic ducts. However, as mentioned in the above chapter, hepatic exploration and, by the same token, intrahepatic biliary duct exploration can be correctly managed only with a linear probe.

4.3.1 The Gallbladder

The gallbladder exploration is simple and quick. The probe is held in direct contact or at a 0.5- to 1-cm distance. In the latter case, it is necessary to pour into the operative field a few deciliters of physiological saline in order to avoid any acoustic window. After placing the probe into a transverse position relative to the gallbladder, the probe is repeatedly moved backward and forward. Two or three successive scannings from the fundus to the neck and to the cystic duct are generally sufficient to provide a good appreciation of the thickness of the wall and of the contents of the gallbladder (Fig. 4.5). The normal wall is thin, less than 3 mm thick. It is echogenic and quite visible on the screen, whereas the bile, in its normal state, is anechogenic. By placing the probe in contact with the superior surface of the liver opposite the cystic fossa, one can also effect longitudinal scanning along the axis of the gallbladder and even visualize it through the hepatic parenchyma (Fig. 4.6). Such an approach is necessary to obtain a precise assessment of the local extension of a gallbladder cancer.

4.3.2 The Common Bile Duct

Exploration of the common bile duct does not provoke any more difficulties than exploration of the accessory biliary apparatus. It requires, however, a little experience on the part of the surgeon. While the technique is being learned, it is recommended that normal anatomic conditions be determined by means of an excellent exposure of the hepatic pedicle. The probe is kept distant from the elements of the hepatic pedicle, while acoustic contact is continuously maintained using physiologic saline. Under visual control, the probe is then placed just over the common bile duct in the middle of its pedicular part, enabling it to be immediately detected on the screen. The section must be transverse. In this way, there is no difficulty in finding the bile duct's section, as well as the sections of other elements of the hepatic pedicle (Fig. 4.7). In its normal state, the common bile duct measures less than 8 mm in diameter; the walls are thin and echogenic, and the contents are anechogenic. The portal vein is situated posteriorly and medial to the common bile duct and measures approximately 16 mm in diameter. The walls of the portal vein are also thin. In its lumen, we can distinguish echoes moving toward the liver that correspond to the flow of portal blood. The hepatic artery, located medial to the bile duct, has approximately the same caliber as the latter. Its pulsations are visible on the screen. This preliminary transverse view of the hepatic pedicle therefore allows good location of all the constituent elements. Keeping the common bile duct in the center of the screen, the probe is moved slowly toward its termination. In this manner, the probe passes anterior to the duodenum and the head of the pancreas. The bile duct, which appeared superficial on the screen, becomes deeper because other elements are interposed between the duct and the probe. It is always difficult to obtain a good view of the bile duct as far as the second part of the duodenum. This is the reason why duodenopancreatic detachment is useful, as it permits nontransverse sections to be performed: in particular, a longitudinal sec-

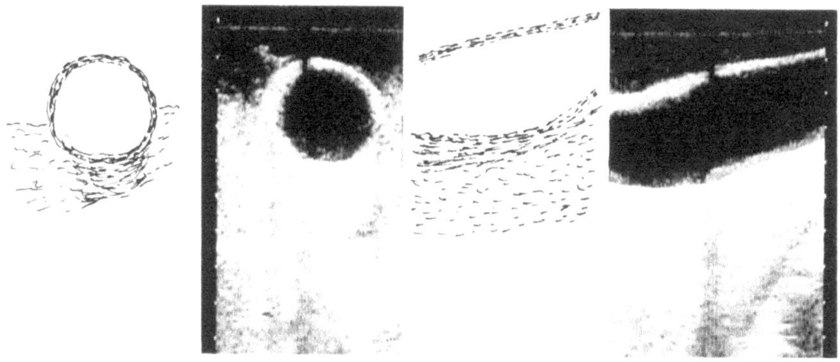

Fig. 4.5. Transverse and longitudinal sections of a normal gallbladder

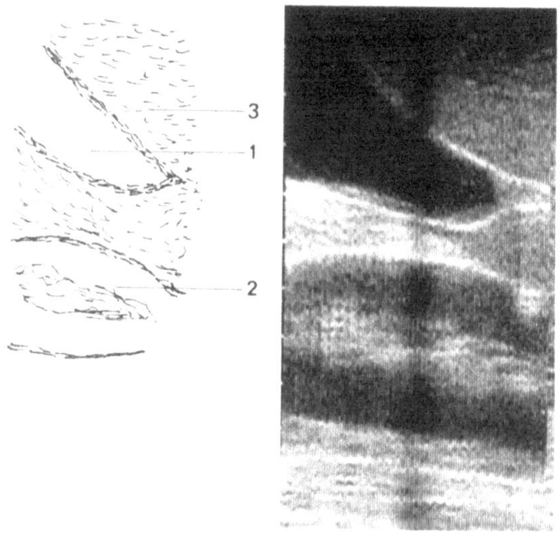

Fig. 4.6. Section of a normal gallbladder through the hepatic parenchyma; *1*, gallbladder; *2*, right kidney; *3*, liver

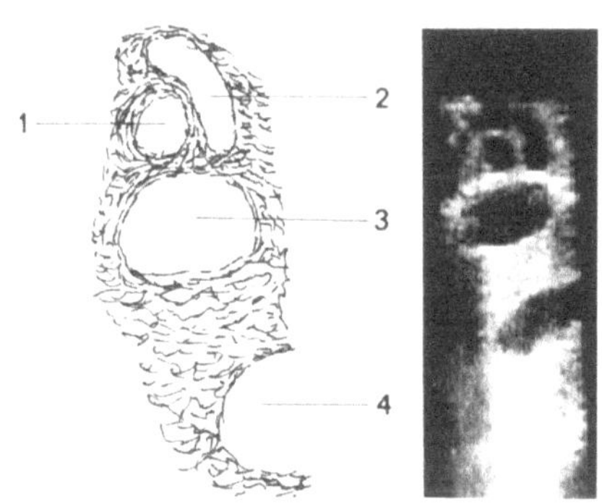

Fig. 4.7. Transverse section of the hepatic pedicle; *1*, common bile duct; *2*, hepatic artery; *3*, portal vein; *4*, inferior vena cava

tion of the common bile duct through the duodenum (Fig. 4.8). This double approach transversely from anterior to posterior, as well as longitudinally from right to left, is often necessary to explore the last few centimeters of the bile duct. It is important to know that it is not absolutely necessary to visualize the bile duct and its lumen as far as the ampulla of Vater. In its normal state, its terminal diameter is very small, so that it is hardly distinguishable on the screen. However, in the presence of lithiasis, the calculi will be visible. Even though the ending of the common bile duct is less visible, sonography is not cholangiography; we must not try to recapture on the sonograph screen what we are used to seeing on the screen of a brilliance amplifier.

Returned to a transverse position, the probe then ascends again to the superior biliary convergence. Do not forget the cystic junction and know how to recognize the image of this meeting point on the screen.

4.3.3 Hepatic Hilum and Intrahepatic Biliary Ducts

The superior biliary convergence and the right and left primary hepatic ducts are explored, starting from the hilum with direct contact of the probe which must always be placed transversely, in contrast to the common bile duct exploration previously performed. In the normal state, in the absence of any dilatation, the primary hepatic ducts are visible in these hilar sections (Fig. 4.9). It is more difficult to locate them when exploring the superior biliary convergence through the parenchyma by placing the probe on the superior surface of the liver (Fig. 4.10). In contrast, the superior biliary convergence is well visualized if the biliary ducts are dilated (Fig. 4.11). From the secondary ducts on, the intrahepatic biliary ducts are not visible. This fact is not important because the aim of sonographic exploration of the intrahepatic bile ducts is not to find normal ducts, but to find dilated ones or intrahepatic lithiases. As a matter of fact dilated biliary ducts are distinctly visible on intraoperative or conventional sonograms. Similarly, stones have sufficiently characteristic acoustic shadows to be detected within the hepatic parenchyma, where it is easy to locate them precisely.

4.3.4 Traps in Exploration

In fact, there are no real anatomical traps in sonographic bile-duct exploration. Sonographic anatomy has to be learned in order to distinguish the different elements of the hepatic pedicle and follow the bile duct from the hilum to its termination. This learning process takes a little while, and errors committed during the training period are principally errors in the identification of these elements. However, certain anatomic anomalies can be unexpected, which is why they have to be kept in mind. The most frequent of these are the termination of the cystic duct on the left side of the common bile duct and the presence of a right hepatic artery arising from the superior mesenteric artery posterior to it. For the same reason, we

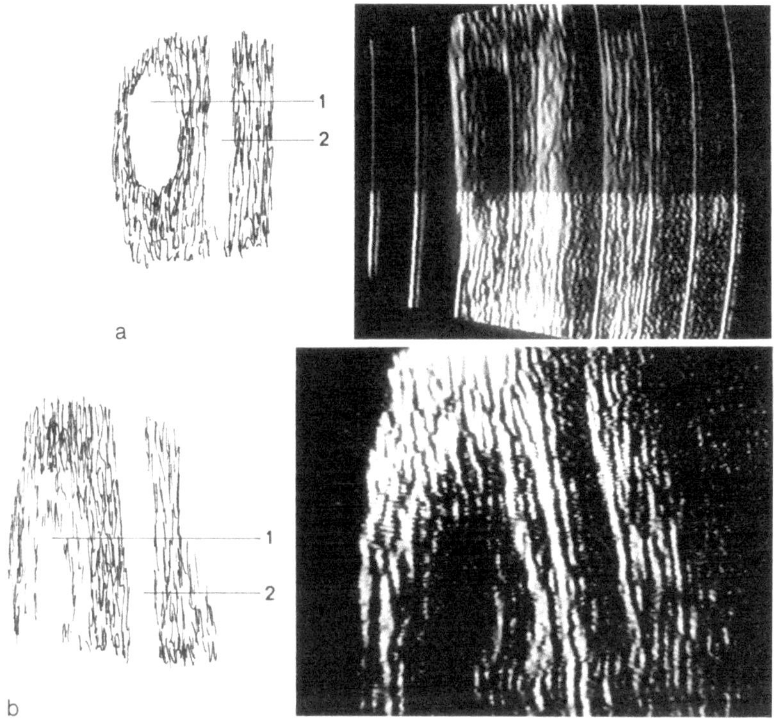

Fig. 4.8 a, b. Longitudinal section of the retroduodenal common bile duct. Such an image of the duodenum can only be obtained when it is filled with fluid; *1*, duodenum; *2*, common bile duct

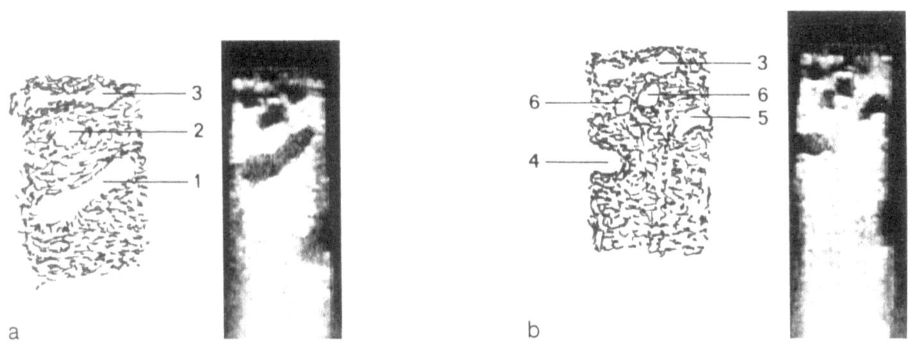

Fig. 4.9 a, b. Transverse section of the porta hepatis. **a** Section through the portal bifurcation with section of the common bile duct and bifurcation of the hepatic artery. **b** Section at a superior level to **a**, showing the right and left portal veins, primary hepatic ducts and bifurcation of the hepatic artery; *1*, portal bifurcation; *2*, common bile duct; *3*, bifurcation of the hepatic artery; *4*, right portal vein; *5*, left portal vein; *6*, primary hepatic ducts

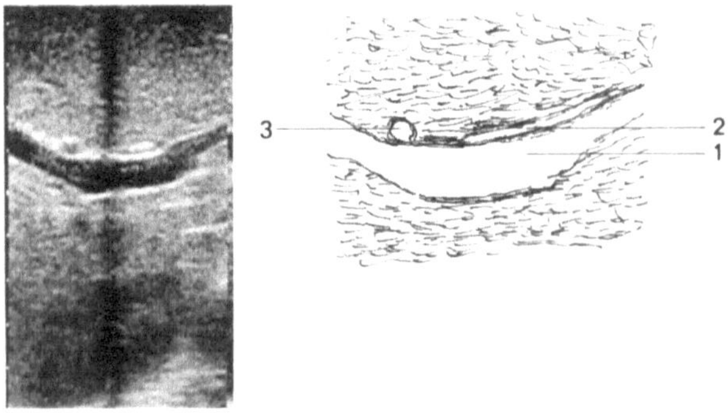

Fig. 4.10. Transverse section of the hepatic pedicle through the hepatic parenchyma; *1*, portal bifurcation; *2*, hepatic convergence; *3*, right branch of the hepatic artery

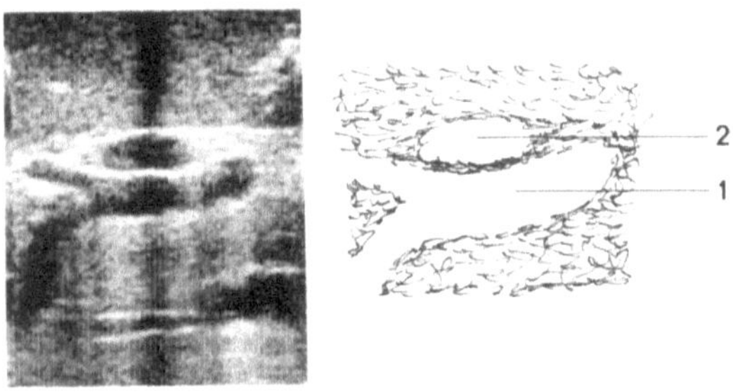

Fig. 4.11. Transverse section of the hepatic pedicle through the hepatic parenchyma in the presence of biliary dilatation; *1*, portal vein; *2*, dilated hepatic bile ducts

advise that, during training time, a good exposure of the hepatic pedicle must be obtained to visualize the biliary duct, in order to place the probe under visual control at its point of contact. The image of a rounded section seen on the screen is in fact the image of the common bile duct. Progressively, one becomes familiar with sonographic anatomy and learns how to detect all the regional structures on the screen directly.

If the anatomic conditions turn out to be more difficult (due to repeated intervention, pericholecystitis, obesity, etc.), and the regional exposure becomes long and delicate, ultrasonography can be used to find the biliary duct within a modified hepatic pedicle. A hepatic artery will be recognized by its caliber, its orientation and, mainly, by its pulsations. The portal vein is recognized by the presence of moving echoes in its lumen. Biliary ducts are often identified by deduction, except in cases of evident abnormality: dilatation, lithiasis, or both. In the case of doubt about the biliary nature of a ductular image, and prior to the commencement of dissection, it is also easy to puncture the duct sonographically to look for bile.

4.4 Biliary Lithiasis

The sonographic image of a biliary stone has a variable appearance. Its echostructure is always hyperechogenic but it appears either rounded or crescentic (Figs. 4.12 and 4.13). Generally, calculi above 0.5 cm in diameter have the shape of a crescent on the sonogram; smaller stones are rounded. Cholesterolic lithiasis is the most common type in the West, but the majority of stones found in the biliary

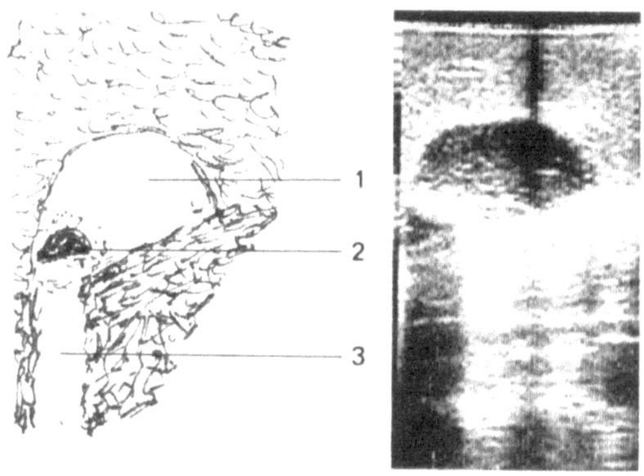

Fig. 4.12. Gallstone: crescentic hyperechogenic image with acoustic shadow; *1*, gallbladder; *2*, stone; *3*, acoustic shadow

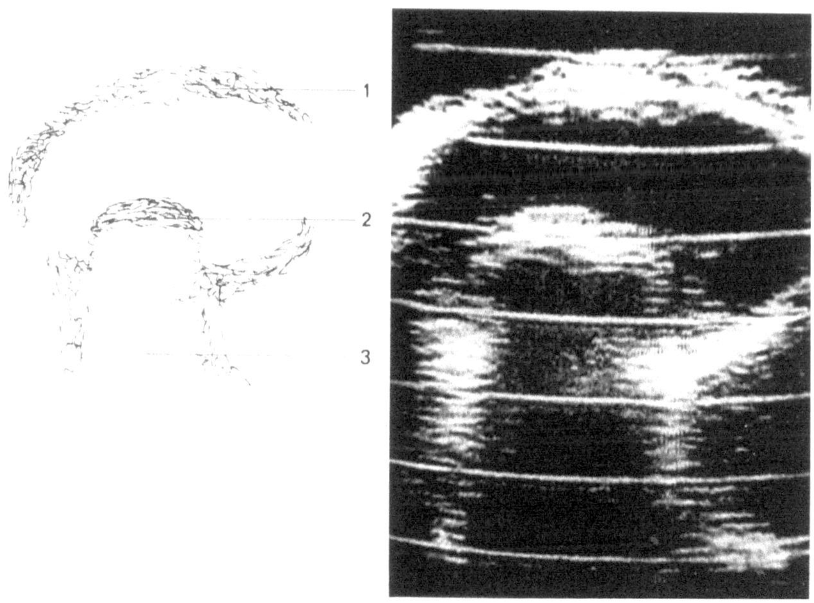

Fig. 4.13. Calculus inside gallbladder with slightly thickened walls; *1*, gallbladder wall; *2*, stone; *3*, acoustic shadow

ducts have a complex constitution. The most usual type of mixed gallstone is the calcified cholesterolic [8]. This explains why the sonographic images of calculi are approximately identical in most cases. The larger the stone, the more easily it is detected. In addition to producing its own image, it absorbs the ultrasound beam. No structures are visible behind it, which is why it is said to produce an acoustic shadow. The presence of this acoustic shadow is an important element contributing to the diagnosis of lithiasis. The association of a hyperechogenic image with a shadow represents without doubt the presence of a calculus in the biliary ducts.

Small calculi and microcalculi theoretically present the same sonographic features. Most cases involve black calculi composed of bilirubin and calcium. The smaller they are, the harder it is to make them evident. They appear as hyperechogenic points, but microlithiases of less than 2 mm diameter have acoustic shadows that are difficult to perceive. In contrast, if several microlithiases are grouped together, we find a series of hyperechogenic points, and the group of microlithiases generates a visible shadow. Sludge or biliary mud is also easy to recognize (Figs. 4.14–4.16). It produces a homogenous echogenic image, but it is not hyperechogenic like calculi are and is without any acoustic shadow.

Can we find any sonographic peculiarities related to the site of lithiasis? There are none; the sonographic patterns are identical whether the site of the lithiasis is the gallbladder or the intra- or extrahepatic biliary ducts. Great difficulties may be encountered in searching for small juxtapapillary calculi (Fig. 4.17) when the anatomic conditions are not favorable (for example, in an obese patient). In the latter case, it is indispensable to effect Kocher's maneuver in order to obtain a transduodenal lateral view of the bile duct's termination, in addition to the transpancreatic transverse scanning procedure.

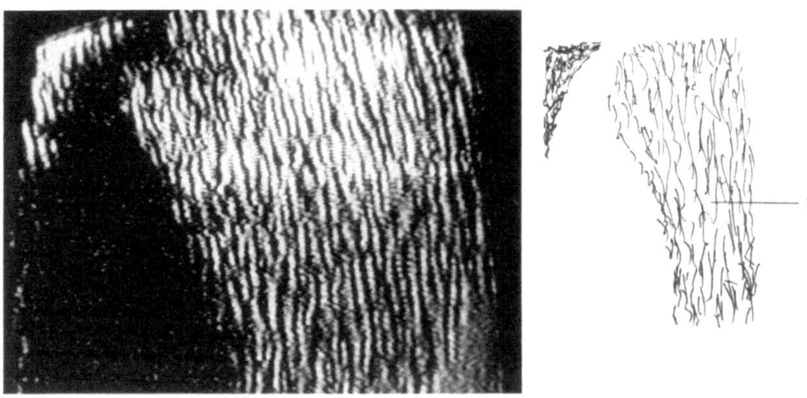

Fig. 4.14. Sludge in gallbladder (hyperechogenic image generating no acoustic shadow); *1*, sludge

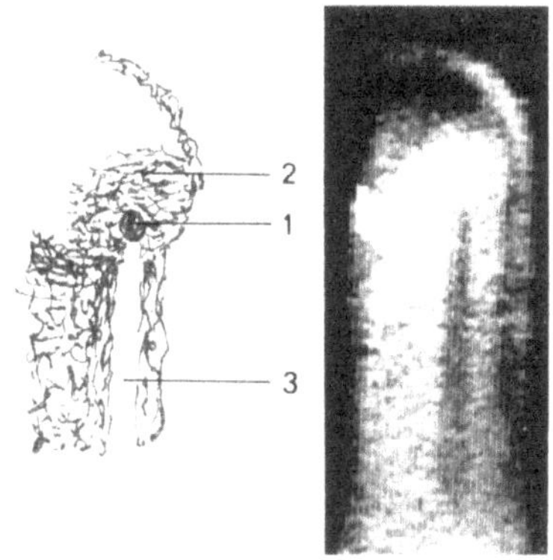

Fig. 4.15. Sludge and gallstone with its acoustic shadow; *1*, stone; *2*, sludge; *3*, acoustic shadow

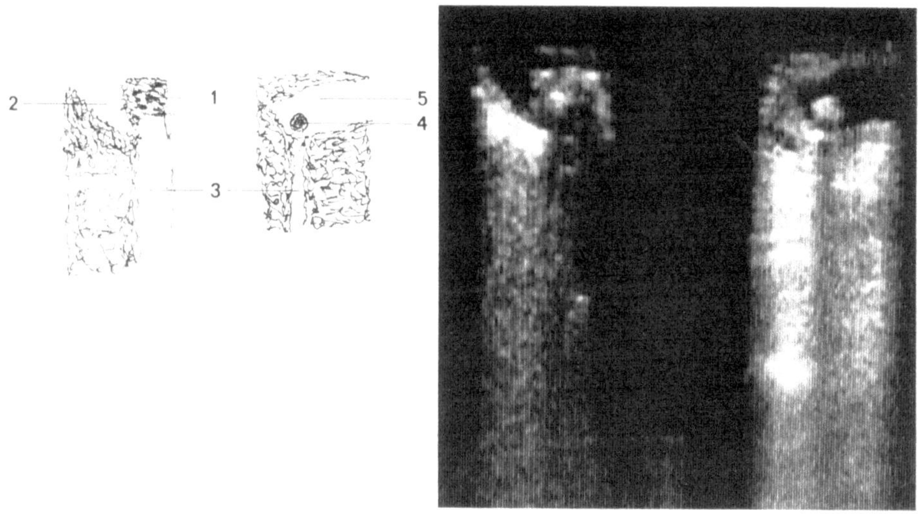

Fig. 4.16. Sludge and calculi inside the gallbladder (*left*), and rounded calculus with its acoustic shadow within the common bile duct (*right*); 1, sludge with calculi; *2*, gallbladder; *3*, acoustic shadow; *4*, stone; *5*, common bile duct

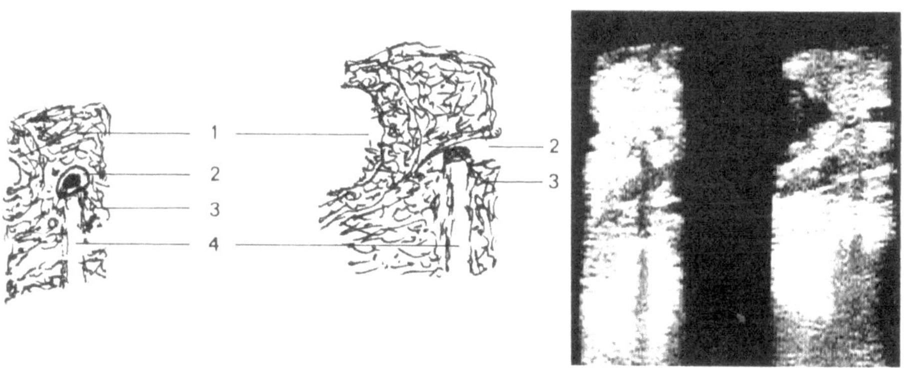

Fig. 4.17. Small (2 mm) juxtapapillary calculus at the termination of the common bile duct; *1*, duodenum; *2*, common bile duct; *3*, stone; *4*, acoustic shadow

4.5 Biliary Tract Stenosis

The information required from intraoperative sonography always concerns the tumor itself, its local extension and the search for hepatic metastases. From a general point of view, tumors of the biliary ducts give an image that suggests thickening of the wall, whose echogenicity is slightly greater than normal. This is not a sufficient sonographic criterion to diagnose malignancy. Thus a cancer of the gallbladder in its initial stage demonstrates parietal thickening the same as in cholecystitis, and cancer of the common bile duct gives an image of stenosis which could well also be of inflammatory origin (Fig. 4.18).

Tumors located at the level of the ampulla of Vater are rather difficult to make evident, as they are small and located within the duodenal wall. They are often associated with upstream pancreatitis, and with common bile duct dilatation or pancreatic duct dilatation, the latter conditions being easier to visualize (Fig. 4.19). Concerning tumors located at the hilum, intraoperative sonography can help to define extension towards the common hepatic duct, the superior biliary convergence, the right and left hepatic ducts, and the secondary biliary convergences. It is also possible to appreciate tumoral extension within the hepatic parenchyma and involvement of other elements of the hilum, particularly the portal vein and the portal bifurcation (Fig. 4.20). Finally, owing to the frequency of their occurrence, we have to know how to detect intrahepatic metastases by ultrasonography.

These cancers of the biliary ducts often cause dilatation of the intrahepatic biliary ducts. During laparotomy any dilated intrahepatic bile duct can be demonstrated, punctured and drained under sonographic guidance. Therefore, external and internal drainage of intrahepatic bile ducts can easily be performed in patients in whom drainage by percutaneous puncture would be difficult and in patients with nonresectable bile duct carcinoma who have obstructed bile ducts [7]. Several new operative procedures have been established in this field. One of these operative procedures consists of establishing drainage from the periphery. After transhepatic puncture of a dilated bile duct, a guide wire is inserted, then replaced by a catheter. This procedure can be monitored clearly by sonography (Fig. 4.21).

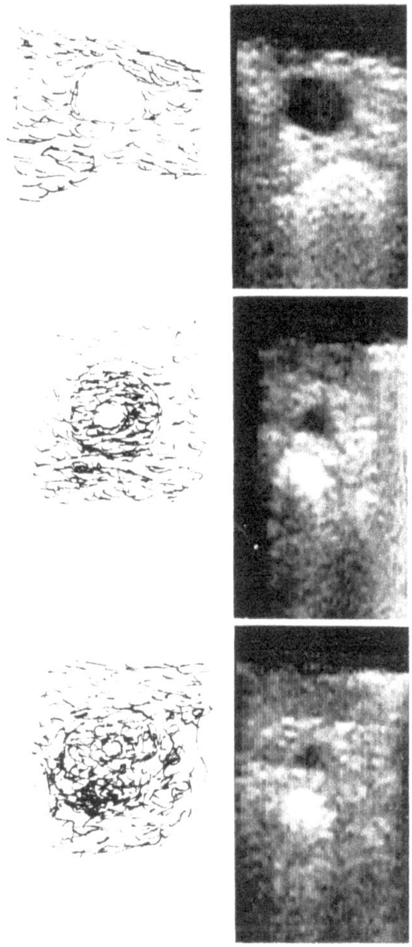

Fig. 4.18. Adenocarcinoma of the common bile duct. Notice the thickening of the wall and the diminution in caliber of the bile duct during up-to-down scanning

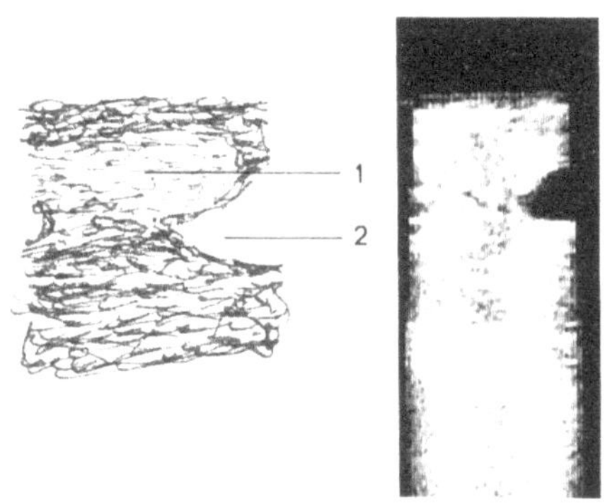

Fig. 4.19. Ampulloma with dilatation of the common bile duct; *1*, ampulloma; *2*, common bile duct

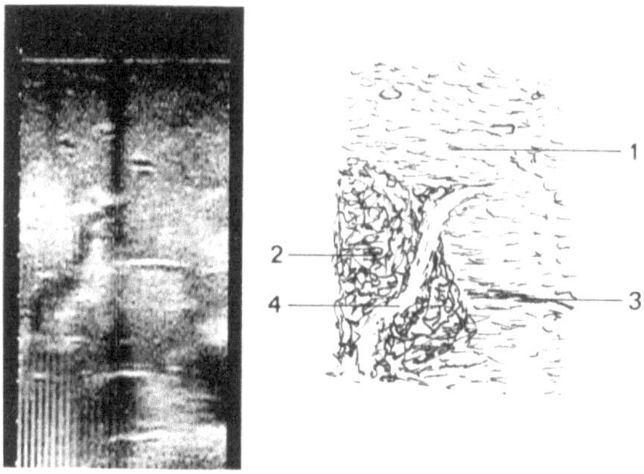

Fig. 4.20. Voluminous cancer of the hilum; *1*, hepatic parenchyma; *2*, tumor; *3*, fissure for ligamentum venosum; *4*, left portal vein

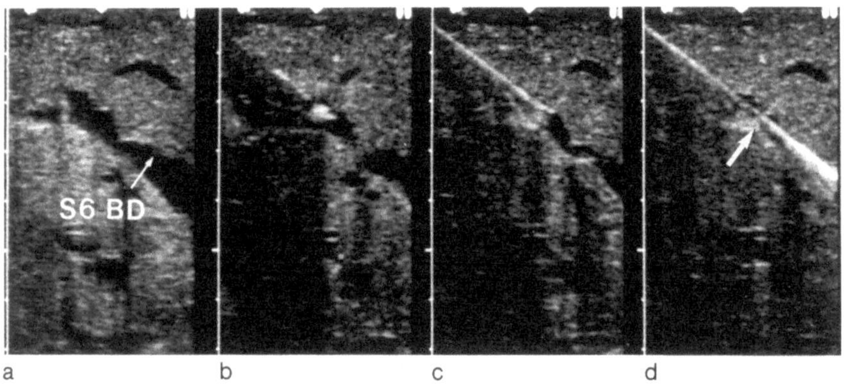

Fig. 4.21 a–d. Puncture of the intrahepatic bile duct and insertion of a drainage tube. **a** The posteroinferior area duct (*S6 - BD*) is extremely dilated due to the carcinoma at the porta hepatis and cholangitis after endoscopic retrograde cholangiography. **b** The peripheral point of the bile duct has been punctured by an 18-gauge teflon-sheathed needle. The tip of the needle is demonstrated in the bile duct. The trunk of the needle casts shadowing behind. **c** The spring guide wire has been inserted from the sheath and the tip of the guide wire is in the sheath. **d** After the guide wire has been advanced as far as possible, the tip of the outer sheath (*arrow*) appears as a change in the reflectivity of the guide wire

4.6 Discussion

As mentioned at the beginning of this chapter cholangiography and, if required, choledochoscopy have for years allowed us to explore the common bile duct during surgery. Surgeons are well trained for these techniques, which, alone or in combination, are generally satisfactory. What then has sonography new to contribute?

The accessory biliary apparatus holds a special position, as it can only be explored by palpation. In this field radiologic opacification offers no advantages in the search for lithiasis or morphologic abnormalities. Palpation is limited. It does not permit recognition of the presence of sludge or small calculi, particularly when the gallbladder is distended, or when its walls are thickened. Consequently, sonography appears to be the only examination permitting accurate exploration and ascertaining the presence of sludge or microlithiasis. The examination is easy, quick, and effective. The images are characteristic enough not to cause confusion.

In most cases, gallbladder calculi are diagnosed prior to intervention, and intraoperative sonography only confirms what is already known. Nonetheless, it may be useful during surgical intervention carried out for a reason other than a biliary problem, in order to determine whether gallstones are present or not, with the aim of preventing acute postoperative cholecystitis. Recently, Herbst et al. [2] drew attention to the advantages of routine intraoperative sonography of the gallbladder for patients who have had surgical intervention for obesity. In this kind of patient, biliary lithiasis is very frequent, with an incidence of up to 38%. Of 55 obese people who underwent surgical intervention (gastric bariatric surgery), nine had gallbladder calculi on palpation, and nine were considered normal, whereas they had demonstrated abnormal sonographic findings. There was only one false-positive sonographic image, which showed density of the wall in the absence of a stone [2].

Gallbladder cancers are mainly encountered in older patients who have had gallstones for a long time and that are often complicated by acute and chronic cholecystitis. Only the initial stages are known to be curable. When the tumor extends through the gallbladder wall to invade the hepatic parenchyma or when hepatic metastases are present, the tumor is known to be incurable. The thickening of the wall itself does not provide any specific sonographic evidence of cancer. It is rather the induration or the rough plaque appearance which warn the surgeon. Only urgently arranged histopathologic examination can establish the diagnosis. In contrast, tumoral extension to the hepatic parenchyma by contiguity and the presence of metastasis are indications of severity that are easy to demonstrate by sonography. In addition, quite often, metastatic nodules are encountered in segments IV and V [3]. Sonographic discovery of hepatic lesions in these segments prior to dissection can assist in determining the indications for exeresis.

The intrahepatic biliary ducts are not spontaneously visible with sonography in their normal state, except for the superior biliary convergence and the primary ducts. Nevertheless, they are clearly visualized by cholangiography. In the case of intrahepatic stones sonography should reveal itself as better than cholangiography, with which intrahepatic calculi sometimes are not detected, due to the absence of opacification of distal biliary ramifications or because of superimposition of images. So, using ultrasound, the hyperechogenic image of the calculus, with its acoustic shadow, is distinctly recognizable within the hepatic parenchyma, even if the biliary ducts are not visible. Such investigation of intrahepatic calculi can only be correctly managed by means of a linear probe. With a sectorial probe it is more difficult. This is the reason why Lane and Coupland found that cholangiography was better for the exploration of the intrahepatic biliary ducts when comparing the advantages of sonography and cholangiography during biliary duct exploration (Table 4.1). They used a sectorial probe, which only allowed them to explore the last 6 cm from the convergence of the intrahepatic ducts [5].

Concerning the investigation of common bile duct stones, we can again refer to the comparative table of Lane and Coupland (Table 4.1). They consider the accuracy of both methods to be similar and the advantages of sonography to be essentially related to the technique of implementation. Its noninvasive character, its feasibility, and its quickness held their attention. Despite their statement, we must specify that a long period of training is required to be able to effect complete sonographic exploration of the common bile duct and to be sure of the interpretation within 3-5 min. During training (first 20 or 30 examinations), the exploration easily requires 20-30 min. Having no certainty about what one is looking at, there must inevitably be association with cholangiography, with which the surgeon is familiar. Furthermore, ultrasound does not expose the patient and the surgical team to radiation. There is a tendency to minimize this problem as it is difficult to determine the iatrogenic effects of this type of irradiation. However, standard exposure under brilliance amplification provides approximately 5000 mR/min. The patient and the whole surgical team receive six times more irradiation during 1 min brilliance amplification than with a simple conventional radiograph [6]. The means of protection employed to reduce this are numerous, and it is necessary to remember the elementary rules of precaution.

More recently, Sigel et al. [9] and Jakimowicz et al. [4] reported two important series comparing ultrasonography with cholangiography in the search for common-bile-duct calculi (Table 4.2). The results are still more or less identical; however, a slight advantage is noted with sonography for the predictive values of positive tests. Nonetheless, as mentioned by Bismuth and Castaing, the radiologic

Table 4.1. Comparison of cholangiography and ultrasonography

	Cholangiography	Ultrasonography
Sensitivity	96%	96%
Specificity	96%	93%
Applicability	88%	100%
Logistics	Acceptable	Excellent
Repeatability	Poor	Excellent
Time required	10-15 min	3-5 min
Learning period	Short	Long
Potential for development	Small	Large
Demonstration of biliary flow	Good	Nil
Intrahepatic pathology	Good	Poor

(From [5])

Table 4.2. Accuracy of intraoperative ultrasonography and intraoperative cholangiography

	Ultrasonography		Cholangiography	
	Sigel et al. [9]	Jakimowicz et al. [4]	Sigel et al. [9]	Jakimowicz et al. [4]
Sensitivity (%)	93.8	89	90.9	86
Specificity (%)	98.6	98	95.4	93
Accuracy (%)	98	96	94.8	91
Predictive value of positive test (%)	91	93	73.2	79
Predictive value of negative test (%)	99	97	98.7	96

exploration technique retains an important function [1]. Cholangiography effected with brilliance amplification, by varying the density of the contrast medium and by making X-ray films at specified times under monitor-screen control, gives better results than three standard radiograms at fixed times. In their series of 523 cases, they obtained with cholangiography: sensitivity in 97.9%, specificity in 99%, negative predictive values in 99.5% and positive predictive values in 92%.

Finally, the performances of cholangiography and sonography are mainly competitive in the field of investigation for common-bile-duct stones. In this field the results can be superposed if cholangiography is effected by means of a brilliance amplifier. This technique is performed under view control with a monitor screen and has the further advantage of providing a dynamic visualization of the passage of contrast medium into the duodenum, which is not the case with ultrasound. Should one give preference to cholangiography for that reason? The matter cannot be brought to a firm conclusion and has to be qualified. In reality both methods are complementary. We must not forget that ultrasonography is the only intraoperative exploratory examination of the gallbladder. The most frequent interventions are for simple gallbladder stones, and in those cases sonography can quickly confirm the presence of gallstones and easily explore the common bile duct. This sonographic exploration is sufficient. It is rapid, reliable and noninvasive. When a more difficult or doubtful case of common-bile-duct calculi reveals itself, it may be useful to associate both examinations or to complete by choledochoscopy the one to which the surgeon is most accustomed. The advantages of sonography in the search for intrahepatic lithiasis have already been emphasized.

In tumor pathology of the common bile duct and superior biliary convergence, sonography appears to be useful. It gives information about the volume of the tumor, the degree of stenosis of the biliary duct and the extension of the tumor upstream, downstream, and toward the neighboring elements.

Cancer of the common bile duct are mostly located at the inferior biliary convergence or lower, in which case it is difficult to distinguish them from exocrine pancreatic adenocarcinomas. There should always be a search for portal vein extension and metastases at the level of the liver. Cancers of the ampulla of Vater form a discrete entity. In 25% of cases there are visceral metastases, mostly hepatic [10], and it is in searching for them that intraoperative sonography has an advantage. Tumors located at the superior biliary convergence have three modes of extension: first, to the intrahepatic biliary ducts, the secondary convergences, and the common hepatic duct; secondly, to the hepatic parenchyma itself; finally, to the regional vascular elements. Sonography permits detection of those different extensions. It also allows dilated intrahepatic ducts to be seen, punctured, and opacified (cholangiography is always indispensable), and, eventually, allows the placement of external or internal drainage. Curative exeresis for cancer of the hilum is now performed, and ultrasound indisputably provides information that completes the intraoperative clinical and radiological examination. It helps the surgeon to determine the possibilities for resection and can also modify the operative strategy.

References

1. Bismuth H, Castaing D (1985) Echographie per-opératoire du foie et des voies biliaires. Flammarion Médecine-Sciences, Paris, France
2. Herbst CA, Mittelstadt CA, Staab EV, Buckwalter JA (1984) Intraoperative ultrasonography evaluation of the gallbladder in morbidly obese patients. Ann Surg (December) 691-692
3. Isman H, Brisard M (1984) L'espoir de guérison des cancers de la vésicule biliaire. Arguments pour une conception nouvelle des stades précoces. J Chir 121: 51-55
4. Jakimowicz JJ, Carol EJ, Jurgens PTHJ (1984) The peroperative use of real-time B-mode ultrasound imaging in biliary and pancreatic surgery. Dig Surg 1: 55-60
5. Lane RJ, Coupland GA (1982) Ultrasonic indications to explore the common bile duct. Surgery 91: 268-274
6. Linos DA, Gray JE, Mellrath DC (1980) Risques d'irradiation du personnel de salle d'opération pendant les cholangiographies. Arch Surg 115: 1431-1433
7. Makuuchi M et al (1980) Internal and external drainage of the intrahepatic bile duct by operative sonography. Tan and Sui 11: 1557-1565
8. Paris J, Salembier Y, Gerard A, Paris JC, Roger J (1977) Les lithiases biliaires. Encycl Med Chir Paris, Foie-Pancréas 10: 7047
9. Sigel B, Machi J, Beitler C, Donahue PE, Bombeck CT, Baker RJ, Duarte B (1983) Comparative accuracy of operative ultrasonography and cholangiography in detecting common duct calculi. Surgery 94: 715-720
10. Vankemmel M, Houcke M, Fontaine JF, Talloen P (1978) Cancers des voies biliaires extrahépatiques. Encycl Med Chir Paris, Foie 10: 7057

5 Ultrasonography of the Pancreas

B. Deixonne, F.-M. Lopez, A. Pissas, B. Sigel

5.1 Introduction

Owing to its solid structure and retroperitoneal location, exploration of the pancreas sometimes proves difficult. Up to now, only radiologic techniques have supplemented the information provided by inspection and palpation. These techniques are: ductular opacification by cholangiography or pancreatography, and vascular opacification by ileoportography. Cholangiography simply allows objective verification of the repercussions of a cephalic lesion on the bile duct. Pancreatography can be difficult to effect in the absence of dilation of the principal pancreatic duct. Ileoportography is an invasive and relatively long examination and is very seldom performed in the end. Apart from the fragmentary nature of the information furnished by these different radiologic techniques, they have the drawback of not providing any data about the parenchymatous structure of the gland. Intraoperative sonography does provide such information and further explores ductular structures and the vascular environment. In this context it can be seen to be an easy, quick, richly informative examination.

5.2 Surgical Anatomy of the Pancreas

A digestive, endocrine and exocrine gland, the pancreas is a deep-seated, central organ, transversely fixed to the anterior aspect of the upper part of the lumbar vertebral column in contact with the retroperitoneal space. Anteriorly, it is covered by the other digestive viscera; posteriorly it conceals the aorta and inferior vena cava.

5.2.1 Descriptive Anatomy

The pancreas is laterally elongated and flattened anteroposteriorly. Classically, it presents a head, a body, and a tail. The head is separated from the body by the neck or isthmus lying between the superior mesenteric vessels inferiorly, and the first part of the duodenum superiorly. Surgeons prefer to refer to the right pancreas or duodenopancreas, and left pancreas or splenopancreas, the isthmus always representing the separating boundary (Fig. 5.1). This concept of pancreatic anatomy is more modern, and corresponds better to morphologic, descriptive, histologic, and embryologic reality.

The normal pancreas is firm, granular, and quite friable in consistency and is of a pinkish white color. Its weight varies with age, being 50-200 g. The organ is smaller in women, increasing in size till the age of 40 years, then undergoing involution from the fifties on. It varies in length from 12-22 cm, being 15 cm on average. The height is approximately 4 cm at the body level, 2.5 cm at the neck level, and 7 cm at the head level. The width of the head is approximately 4 cm, its thickness varying between 1.5 and 2 cm. The pancreas is remarkably fixed. It is adherent on the right side to the posterior layer of the mesoduodenum and on the left side to the posterior mesogastrium. Only the tail is mobile within the splenopancreatic ligament. Variations occur, particularly retention of the pancreatic division due to failure of fusion of the ventral and dorsal embryologic primordia. An annular pancreas is due to failure of rotation of the ventral primordium around the duodenum. Sometimes an aberrant or supernumerary pancreas may be encountered in the peritoneal folds surrounding the stomach or the small intestine.

5.2.2 Pancreatic Ducts

The ducts convey the exocrine secretions of the pancreas toward the duodenum. The main pancreatic duct (Wirsungs' duct) is rectilinear in the tail and body. At the neck level it descends obliquely to the right describing a double curve like an italic *S;* the superior curve is concave to the left and inferiorly, the inferior curve is concave to the right and superiorly. In section, the pancreatic duct is strictly axial at the tail level. It slightly approaches the anterior surface of the organ at the body level, equidistant from the superior and inferior borders. In contrast, at the head level, it is located in a posterior plane. Its diameter increases from left to right, from 2 to 3 mm. Its termination is constricted. It receives multiple thin afferents, which are quite regularly distributed and arranged like the legs of a millipede. It terminates in the second part of the duodenum at the major duodenal papilla, to-

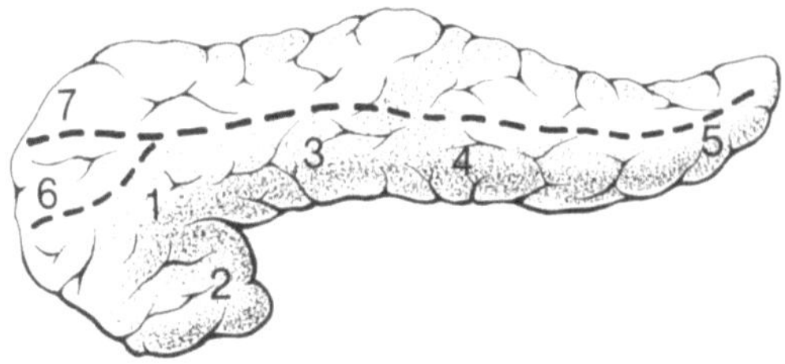

Fig. 5.1. Morphology of pancreas. The right part of the pancreas comprises the head of the pancreas (*1*) and the uncinate process (*2*). *3*, neck. The left part of the pancreas comprises the body (*4*) and the tail (*5*). The *interrupted lines* represent ducts: *6*, principal pancreatic duct (Wirsung's duct); *7*, accessory pancreatic duct (Santorini's duct)

gether with the termination of the common bile duct, with which it has a common inflow into the ampulla of Vater. Variations in this classical pattern occur.

The accessory pancreatic duct (duct of Santorini) drains the anterior surface of the head. Smaller than the main duct, it arises at the junction of the two curves described by the main duct within the head of the pancreas. It is directed superiorly and to the right, describing a concavity inferiorly and to the right. It is anterior to the main duct, and opens into the duodenum halfway between the genu superius and the major duodenal papilla, onto the minor duodenal papilla.

The variations of the pancreatic ducts are numerous and derive from different modalities of embryologic development. There may be an absence of the junction of the two ducts, an absence of one or both ducts, or variations in the level of junction of the ducts.

5.2.3 Vessels

The pancreatic arteries belong to two vascular territories and to a regional supply system (arcus pancreaticoduodenalis anterior, posterior and prepancreaticus). The head of the pancreas is enclosed by its arterial arcades. They represent an anastomotic system between the coeliac trunk and the superior mesenteric artery by means of the gastroduodenal artery above, and the first jejunal arteries below. This anastomosis can ensure the complete substitution of one of the vascular territories by means of the other. The anatomical disposition of the arteries is such that the anastomosis between the two regional vascular systems seems to be direct. The arterial vascularization of the body and tail of the pancreas depends on the splenic artery and the transverse pancreatic artery. The latter comes from the dorsal pancreatic artery and anastomoses with the cephalic arteries. The dorsal pancreatic artery vascularizes the neck of the pancreas.

The venous drainage of the head is performed by arches arranged in an identical manner to the arterial arches but less systematized. The posterior superior pancreaticoduodenal arch flows directly into the portal trunk. The anterior and inferior pancreaticoduodenal arches flow into the superior mesenteric vein via the intermediation of Henle's gastrocolic trunk (i.e., the union of the right gastroepiploic, the anterior pancreaticoduodenal and the right colic veins). The venous drainage of the left side of the pancreas is reliant on the splenic vein, which is a tributary of the portal vein, and on the inferior pancreatic vein, which flows into the superior mesenteric vein posterior to the isthmus.

The lymphatic vessels and their zones of drainage are difficult to systematize, as intraparenchymatous anastomoses are numerous between the anterior and posterior surfaces, as well as between the right and the left sides of the pancreas. It appears that there are two preferential right and left lymphatic streams, with the isthmus as an apparent frontier. The lymphatic collectors terminate in node relays, these nodes being few in number. The posterior lymphatic stream in particular traverses only a single node before reaching the central periaorticocaval nodes, the third relay, via the right and left retropancreatic processes. The short distances involved and the small number or absence of nodes explains the rapid metastasis of malignant tumors of the pancreas.

5.2.4 Relations

Within the duodenopancreatic recess, the pancreas is related to the duodenum, the common bile duct, the arteries, and the veins (Fig. 5.2). Let us simply recall a few points:

The common bile duct penetrates the parenchyma of the pancreatic head, going obliquely inferiorly, anteriorly, and to the right. The pancreas forms a depressed groove or a tunnel around it.

Concerning the arteries, we remember that in 17% of cases there exists a right hepatic artery arising from the superior mesenteric artery. Near its origin, the right hepatic artery makes its way into the right retroportal process. It is situated in the pancreatic fossa, intimately associated with the organ, and accompanying it during Kocher's maneuver.

The venous relations are the most important ones; posterior to the pancreas are the tributaries and the origin of the portal trunk. The splenic vein, coming from the spleen, crosses the anterior surface and the superior border of the tail of the pancreas to follow a course on the posterior surface inferior to the artery. The inferior mesenteric vein arrives at the duodenojejunal angle and slips to the posterior side of the pancreas to join the splenic vein and form the splenomesenteric trunk. The superior mesenteric vein passes through the anterior aspect of the uncinate process and ascends to the posterior side of the isthmus to receive the splenomesenteric trunk from the left side. The portal vein is formed in this manner at a variable level. An actual layer of pancreatic parenchyma can surround the vein and cover part or all of the posterior surface.

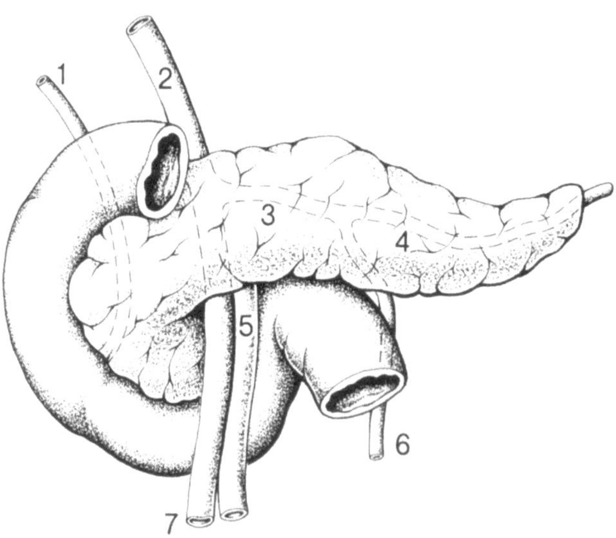

Fig. 5.2. Contents of pancreatic sheath. *1*, common bile duct (ductus choledochus); *2*, portal vein; *3*, junction of splenic vein and inferior mesenteric vein; *4*, splenic vein; *5*, superior mesenteric artery; *6*, inferior mesenteric vein; *7*, superior mesenteric vein

Through the duodenopancreatic recess, the pancreas is related anteriorly to the insertion of the transverse mesocolon. It crosses the inferior part of the head and neck horizontally, following the inferior border of the pancreatic body, and defines a submesocolic and a supramesocolic segment. Superior to the insertion of the transverse mesocolon, the important relations are the stomach and the first part of the duodenum by means of the omental bursa.

The posterior relations are different for the right and the left sides of the pancreas. The duodenopancreas is adherent to the visceral fascia (Fig. 5.3) which covers posteriorly the retroperitoneal space itself. This is Treitz's fascia. It is easy to detach the duodenopancreas and separate the posterior plane by Kocher's maneuver. The duodenopancreas is free of peritoneum on its posterior aspect, and through Treitz's fascia it is closely related to the inferior vena cava, covering at this level the terminations of both renal veins and of the right gonadal vessels.

The splenopancreas adheres to the posterior abdominal wall through the fusion of the dorsal mesogastrium with the visceral fascia. This is Toldt's fascia. The body and the tail of the pancreas are closely related to the left crus of the diaphragm, the left renal pedicle and the left kidney. Medial to the superior pole of the kidney the pancreas covers the inferior half of the anterior surface of the left suprarenal gland.

In the midline, at the isthmus level, the pancreas is in direct contact with the insertion of the primary dorsal mesentery of the aorta. Superior to the superior border of the pancreas, the celiac trunk arises, flanked by the two celiac ganglia. At the first lumbar vertebral level, covered by the posterior aspect of the pancreatic isthmus, the superior mesenteric artery takes its origin, describing an arch as far as the inferior border of the isthmus. At each side of its origin are the superior mesenteric ganglia. They are connected with the ganglia above by numerous fibers. Inferior to the origin of the superior mesenteric artery, the aorta is crossed by the left renal vein, which passes through the angle formed by the aorta and the superior mesenteric artery. The latter crosses anterior to the left renal vein (Fig. 5.4).

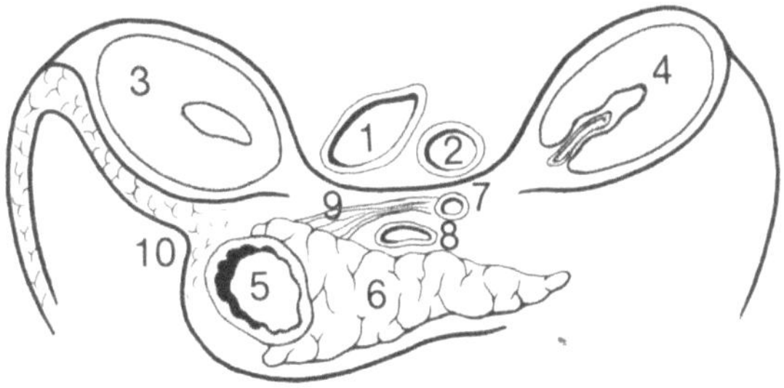

Fig. 5.3. Transverse section through pancreas. *1,* inferior vena cava; *2,* abdominal aorta; *3,* right kidney; *4,* left kidney; *5,* second part of duodenum; *6,* pancreas; *7,* superior mesenteric artery; *8,* portal vein; *9,* retroportal process; *10,* retropancreatic fascia

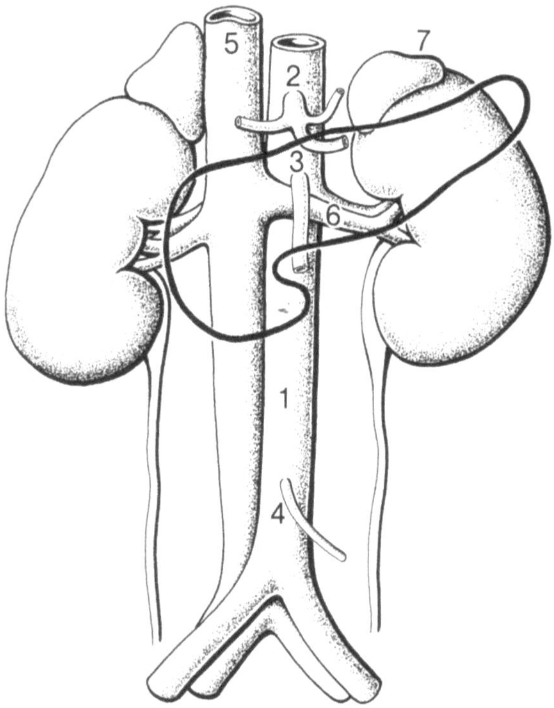

Fig. 5.4. Posterior relations of the pancreas. *1*, abdominal aorta; *2*, celiac trunk; *3*, superior mesenteric artery; *4*, inferior mesenteric artery; *5*, inferior vena cava; *6*, left renal vein; *7*, left kidney and suprarenal gland

5.3 Technical Exploration and Ultrasound Findings

Sonographic exploration of the pancreas does not require any special approaches. They are those of pancreatic surgery, i.e., bisubcostal or median celiotomy allowing good exposure of the gland. We give preference to the bisubcostal incision, as it provides a wider field, useful especially in oncologic surgery.

As with manual exploration, it is necessary to open the omental bursa by sectioning the gastrocolic ligament or by coloepiploic detachment. Although not absolutely indispensable, it is better to free the anterior side of the pancreatic head, and unhook the duodenopancreas by Kocher's maneuver. The pancreas and all its segments are then readily accessible and their exploration is facilitated.

Owing to the thinness of the gland and for good vision of its superficial planes, the probe must not be placed in direct contact with the gland but kept 1 cm distant from its surface. To obtain an acoustic window, it is enough to pour a few deciliters of physiologic saline solution into the operative field. For the same effect one can place a water bag over the probe.

The exploration starts at the isthmus level by placing the probe in a longitudinal and slightly oblique position in order to find the essential landmark, the mesentericoportal venous axis. We thus obtain a longitudinal section of the isthmus, with the portal vein in sagittal section, and the main pancreatic duct in transverse section (Fig. 5.5). Normally, the pancreas is not very thick at this level, ranging between 13 and 15 mm. The caliber of the portal vein is 16 mm. The main pancreatic duct, which crosses anterior to the portal vein, has a median diameter of 2.5 mm. In a more posterior plane, one can easily identify the inferior vena cava in sagittal section. It appears pulsatile, of 20 mm caliber, and varies with the respiratory movements.

The exploration will be effected to the left, then to the right, by longitudinal or transverse sections. The vascular elements are always the easiest to identify. They are the best landmarks. They are bordered by a thin echogenic strip, and echoes

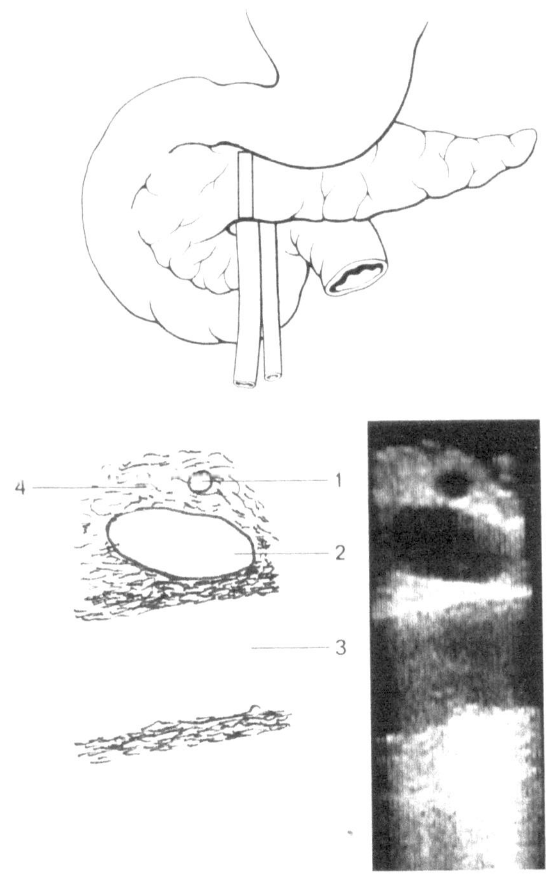

Fig. 5.5. Longitudinal section of pancreatic isthmus. *1*, principal pancreatic (Wirsung's) duct; *2*, portal vein; *3*, inferior vena cava; *4*, pancreatic isthmus. The *shaded rectangle* represents the probe

corresponding to the blood flow circulate in the lumen. Toward the left, the spleno-mesenteric trunk and the splenic vein have diameters of 5-12 mm. At the corporeocaudal level, a longitudinal section through the body and tail shows the pancreatic parenchyma, whose thickness varies between 10 and 20 mm, the main pancreatic duct having here a caliber of less than 2 mm, and the splenic vein on the posterior aspect of the pancreas (Fig. 5.6). In a transverse section of the neck and the body we can identify all the vascular elements related to the posterior surface: the portal vein, the superior mesenteric artery, the left renal vein, and posterior to it, the aorta (Figs. 5.7 and 5.8). The superior mesenteric artery is posterior and medial to the portal vein: its caliber is 3-4 mm, and it appears pulsatile. Its wall is not distinct from the other vascular elements. This vascular crossroad is an excellent landmark, because, starting from it, the mesenteric artery can be followed along its entire retropancreatic course to its aortal origin (Fig. 5.9).

Exploration of the right pancreas also has to be carried out using a succession of longitudinal and transverse sections. The head is 20 mm thick. In the normal state, the common bile duct is not always easily made prominent. Its caliber throughout its pancreatic course is constricted to 2-3 mm; its course is short and its location is posterior.

In a transverse section close to the superior border of the pancreas, one can distinguish the portal vein, the gastroduodenal artery, and the common bile duct (Fig. 5.10). In a transverse section on the lower part of the cephalic region, we again find the main pancreatic duct. Superior to this duct is the termination of the common bile duct (Fig. 5.11). We are at the level of the ampulla of Vater.

A normal pancreas appears moderately echogenic on the sonographic screen. It is sometimes difficult to visualize well, and for this reason it may be necessary to vary the gain and the adjustments of dynamic amplification. The thinness of the pancreas and its average echogenicity are the reasons why exploration is difficult in the normal state. Similarly, the fine caliber of the ductular elements sometimes entails arduous investigation. Only vascular elements can be located and identified perfectly. In contrast, as soon as a lesion modifies the sonographic structure

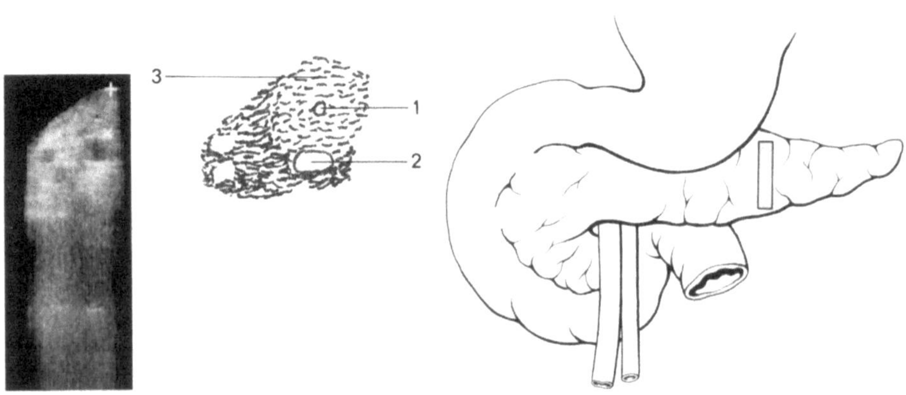

Fig. 5.6. Longitudinal section of pancreatic tail. *1*, principal pancreatic (Wirsung's) duct; *2*, splenic vein; *3*, pancreas. The *shaded rectangle* represents the probe

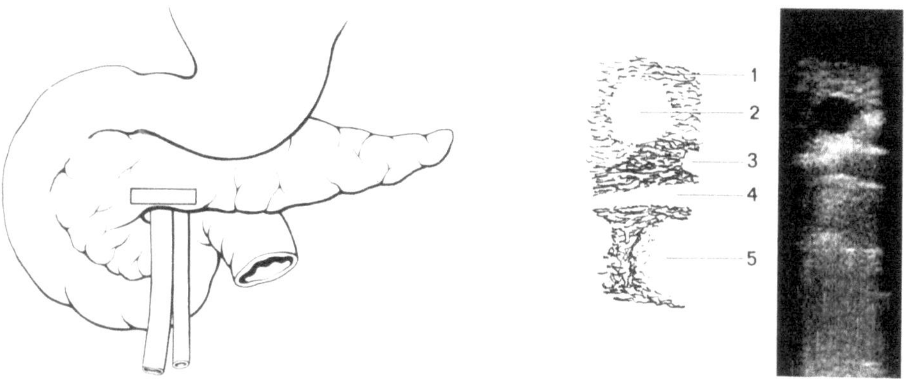

Fig. 5.7. Transverse section of pancreatic body. *1*, pancreas; *2*, superior mesenteric vein; *3*, superior mesenteric artery; *4*, left renal vein; *5*, aorta. The *shaded rectangle* represents the probe

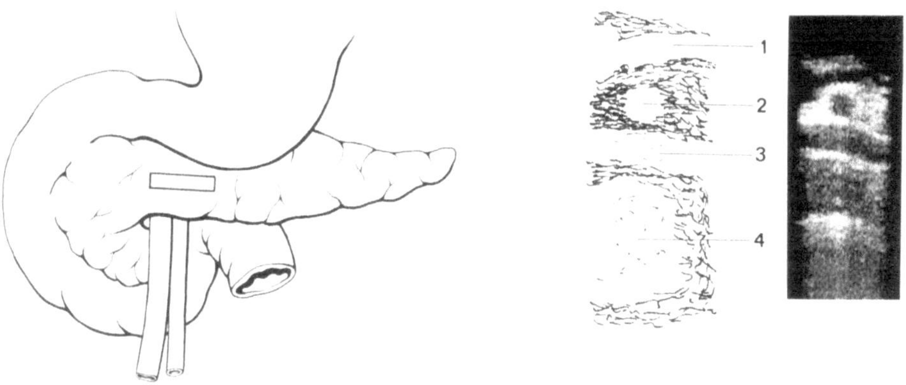

Fig. 5.8. Transverse section of pancreatic body (vascular landmarks). *1*, portal vein and splenomesenteric trunk; *2*, superior mesenteric artery; *3*, left renal vein; *4*, aorta. The *shaded rectangle* represents the probe

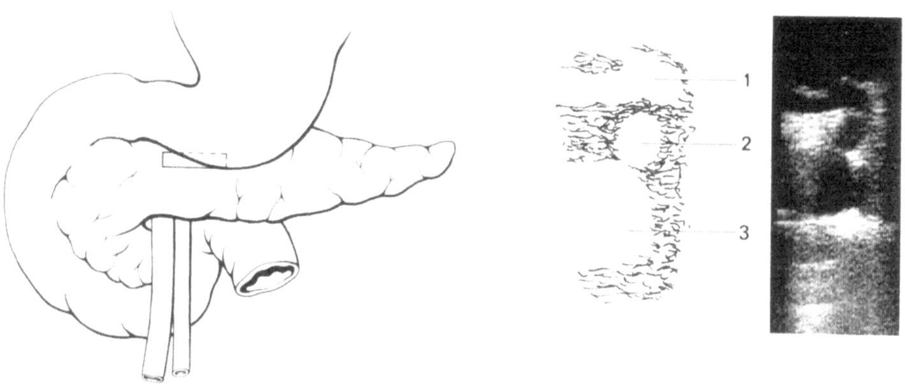

Fig. 5.9. Transverse section of pancreatic body (vascular landmarks). *1*, splenomesenteric trunk; *2*, superior mesenteric artery; *3*, aorta. The *shaded rectangle* represents the probe

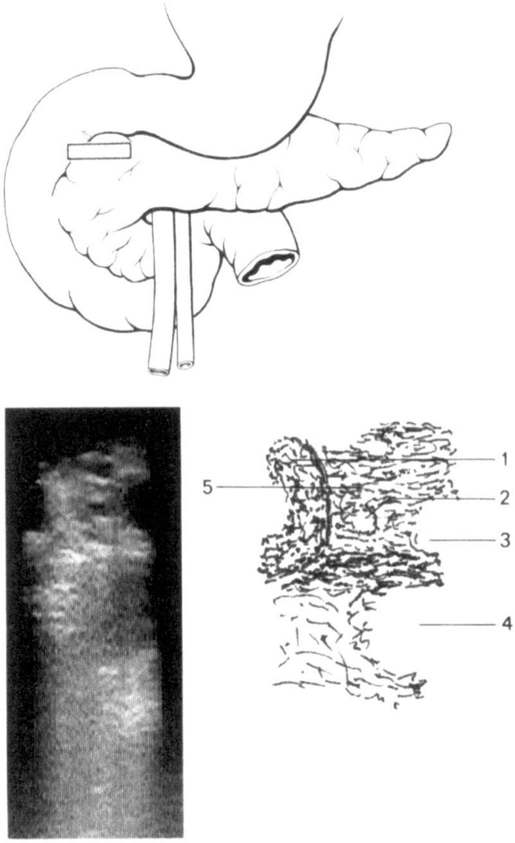

Fig. 5.10. Transverse section of pancreatic head. *1*, duodenum; *2*, common bile duct; *3*, portal vein; *4*, inferior vena cava; *5*, pancreas. The *shaded rectangle* represents the probe

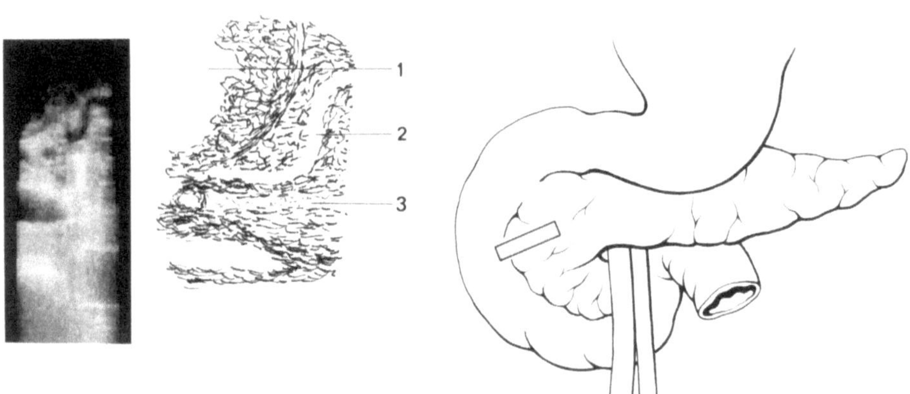

Fig. 5.11. Oblique transverse section of pancreatic head, showing chronic pancreatitis after left pancreatectomy. *1*, duodenum; *2*, common bile duct; *3*, principal pancreatic (Wirsung's) duct, in which a metallic needle is placed. The *shaded rectangle* represents the probe

of the parenchyma, invades or displaces the vessels or has repercussions on the ductular elements such as stenoses with upstream dilatations, this is more easily seen on examination.

5.4 Chronic Pancreatitis and Pancreatic Cysts

Chronic pancreatitis is not a rare disease. Essentially of ethylic origin, its onset appears as a sclerosis of the parenchyma (Figs. 5.12-5.14). Later on, protein-linked calcium precipitation into the excretory ducts occurs, leading to calculus formation in the ducts, ductules, and main pancreatic duct [6]. The lesions are either localized in part of the gland, or are (more often) diffuse. Even in the latter case, there is always predominant involvement of the right or left pancreas. Sometimes, the lesions have a nodular or multinodular nature impossible to distinguish sonographically from exocrine pancreatic cancer.

a
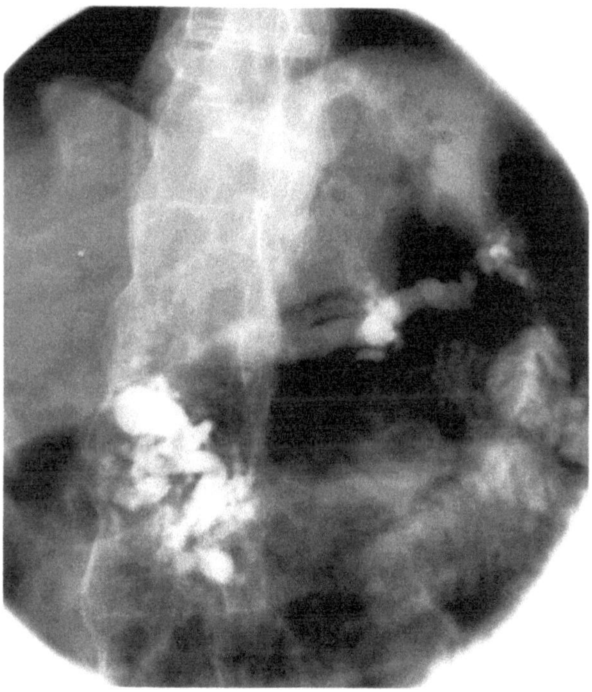

Fig. 5.12a-e. Diffuse chronic pancreatitis of ethylic origin. **a** Preoperative pancreatography: cystic dilatation of several ductules, particularly in the head of the pancreas with irregular principal pancreatic duct. **b** Intraoperative sonography: we find a dilated and irregular principal pancreatic duct. In addition, there is a rounded calculus with a small acoustic shadow. The pancreatic parenchyma is generally hyperechogenic. *1*, pancreas; *2*, principal pancreatic duct; *3*, stone; *4*, splenomesenteric trunk; *5*, acoustic shadow. **c** Intraoperative pancreatography: opacification of the principal pancreatic duct in its caudal and corporal portions. **d** Intraoperative cholangiography: stenosis of the termination of the common bile duct. **e** Schematic representation of the location of pancreatic calculi (continued on p. 120)

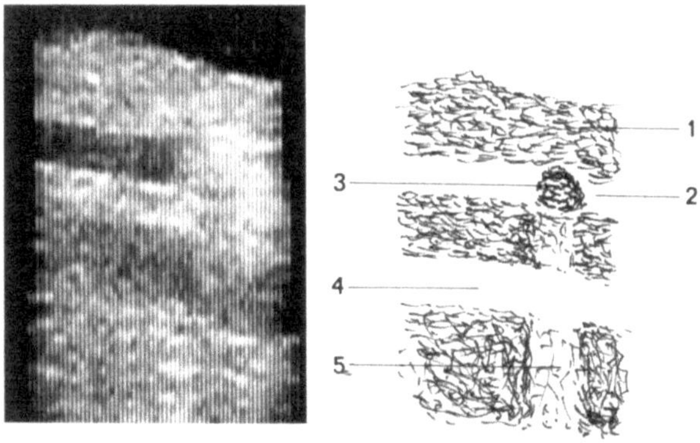

b

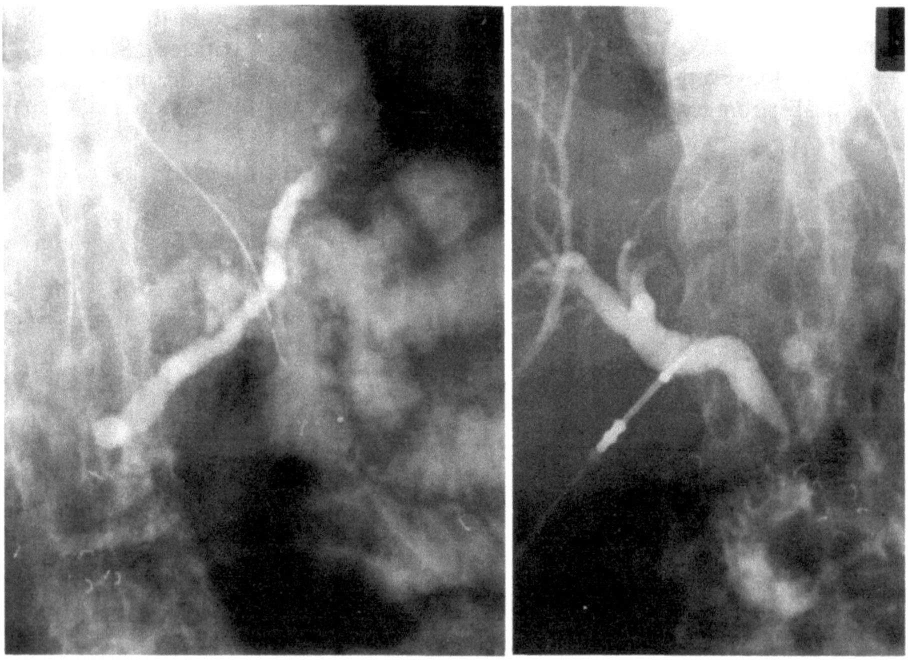
c,d

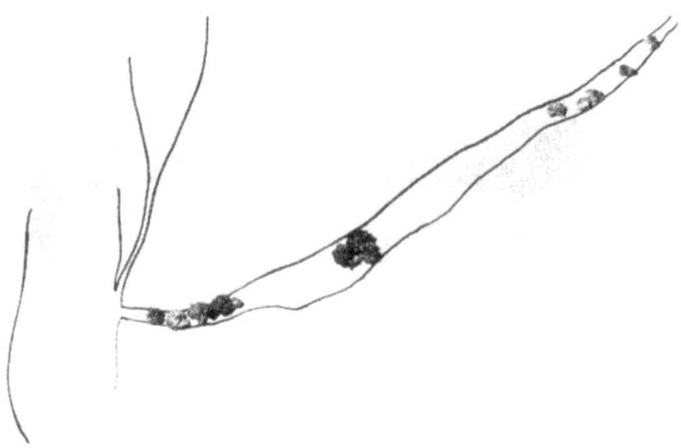
e

Fig. 5.12 b–e (continued)

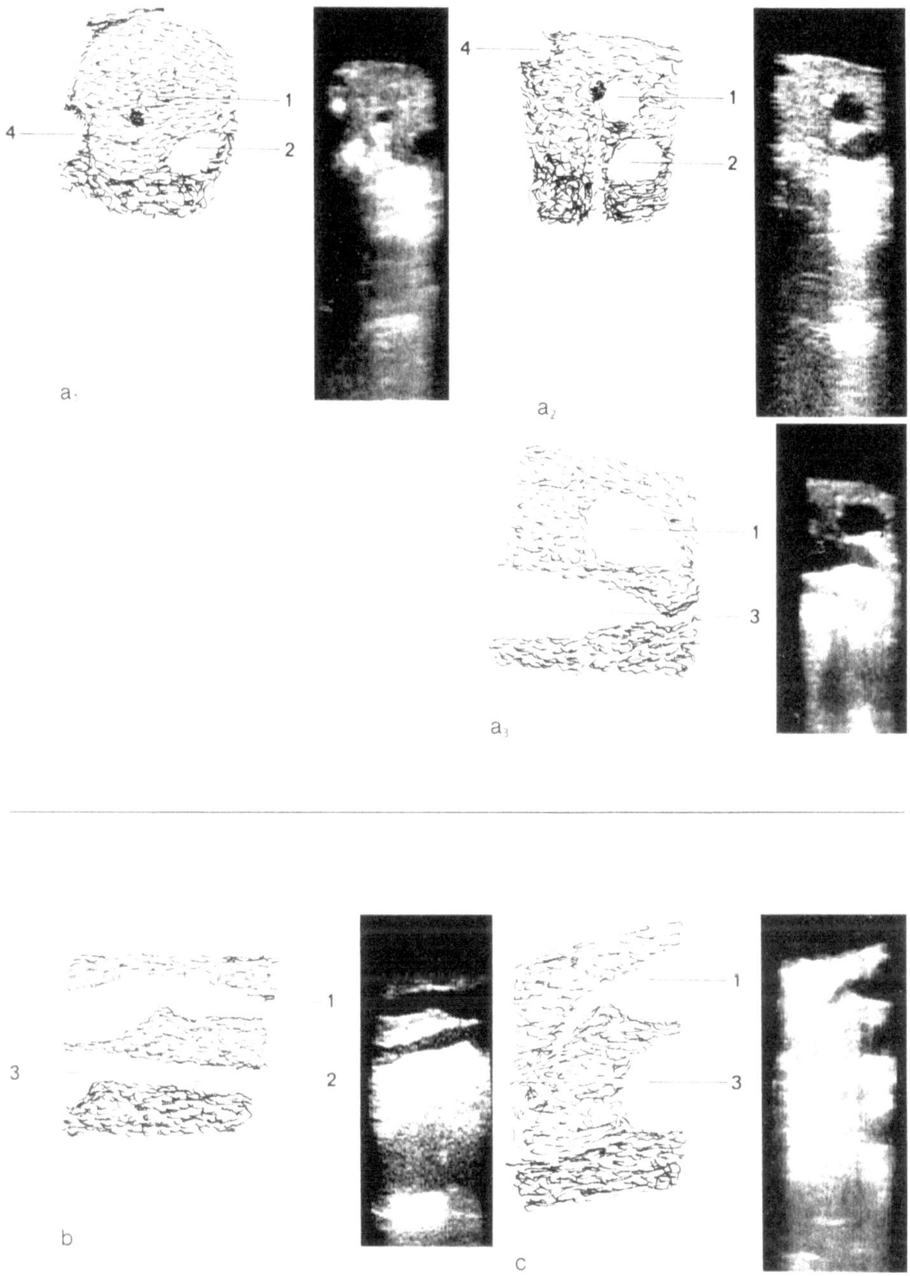

Fig. 5.13 a–c. Diffuse chronic pancreatitis of ethylic origin. **a** Longitudinal sections at the tail level (**a_1**), at the body level (**a_2**), and at the level of the pancreatic isthmus (**a_3**). Notice the change in caliber of the principal pancreatic duct, and thick calcification in the corporal section. There is no intraductular calculus. **b** Transverse section at the body level, showing irregular dilatation of the principal pancreatic duct. **c** Transverse section at the head level. The principal pancreatic duct ends in significant stenosis. In the posterior part, the portal vein is visible; *1*, principal pancreatic duct; *2*, splenic vein; *3*, portal vein; *4*, splenic artery

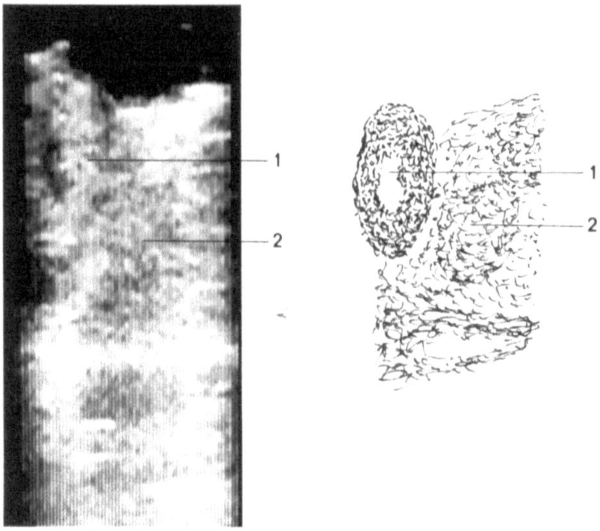

Fig. 5.14. Ethylic chronic pancreatitis predominantly involving the left pancreas; transverse section of the head passing below the termination of the principal pancreatic duct. The sonographic appearance is not very abnormal; *1*, duodenum; *2*, head of pancreas

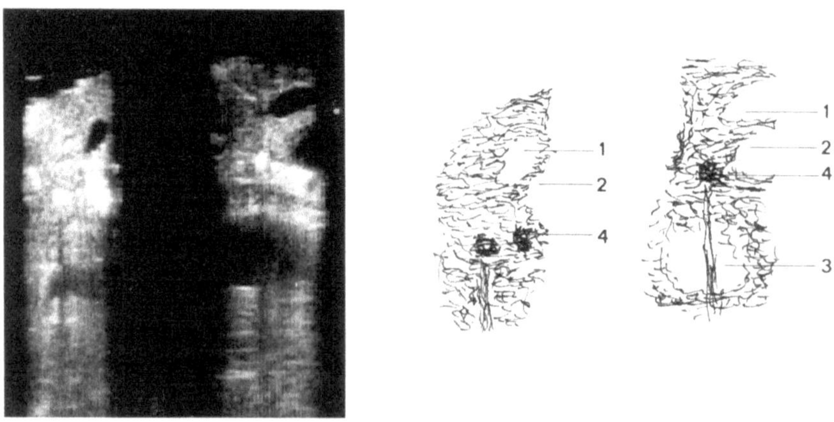

Fig. 5.15. Chronic pancreatitis predominantly involving the head of the pancreas; the principal pancreatic duct is slightly dilated (6 mm). There are clearly distinguishable calcic deposits in the parenchyma; *1*, principal pancreatic duct; *2*, portal vein; *3*, inferior vena cava; *4*, calcic deposits

Fig. 5.16 a–c. Pseudocyst of the pancreas with pancreatitis. **a** Preoperative computed tomography. **b** Intraoperative ultrasonography: longitudinal section showing the absence of communication between cyst (*C*) and main pancreatic duct (*W*). **c** Opacification of the cyst confirms the absence of communication with the principal pancreatic duct

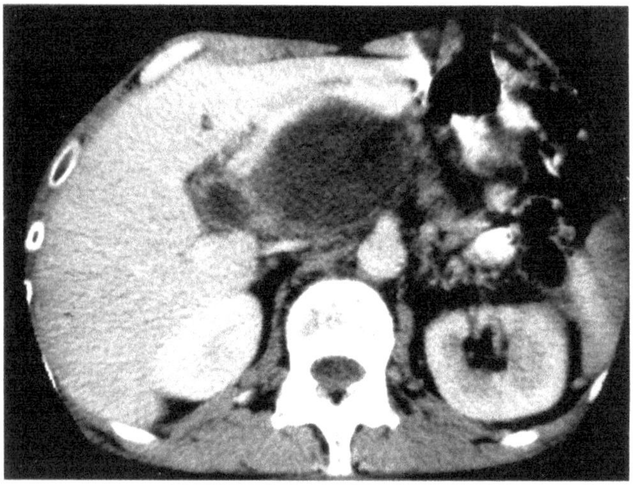

a

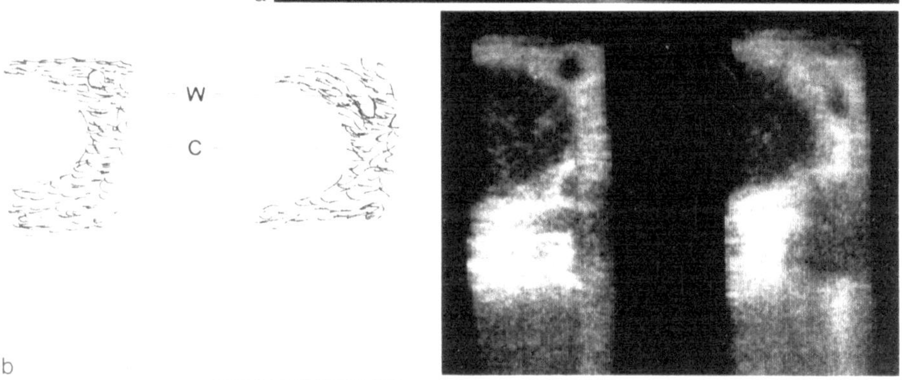

b

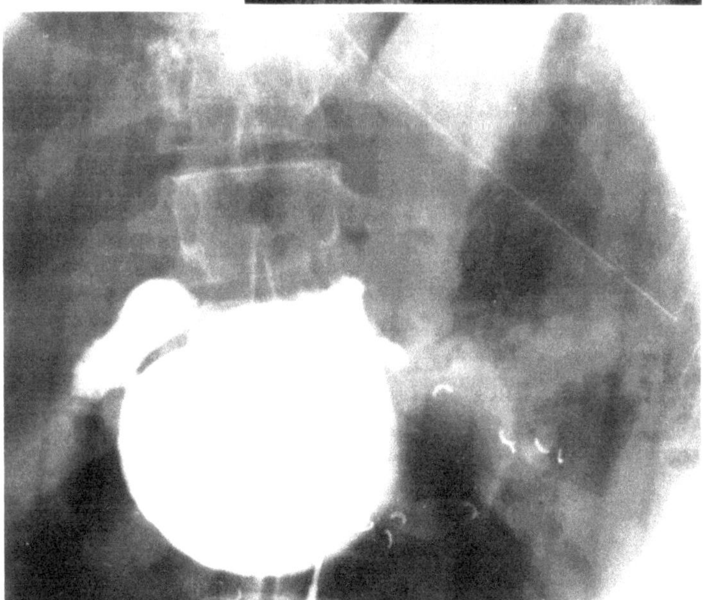

c

All the glandular alterations are visible with ultrasound. Increase in pancreatic volume is usual, and its dimensions are easy to determine. The parenchyma appears heterogeneous, but essentially hyperechogenic: the echogenicity varies in relation to the severity of the lesion. This hyperechogenicity is shown by many brilliant points or lines separated by fine anechogenic lattices corresponding to ductules. The points and lines correspond to sclerotic zones and to calcic precipitations.

The main pancreatic duct is usually dilated (Fig. 5.15). Again, we find modifications in its caliber, and sometimes lithiases. The latter differ in sonographic appearance from biliary lithiases, which are often more voluminous and form lunar crescents with well-marked acoustic shadows. Pancreatic calcic calculi are easily seen to have rounded images with a faint acoustic shadows.

Cystic dilatations or pseudocysts are also very easy to make evident (Fig. 5.16). The content of cysts is on the whole anechogenic, but we very often find echoes corresponding to necrotic fragments. Apart from its advantages for evaluating correlations between cysts, ultrasonography allows the thickness of the walls to be measured, which is useful when an internal bypass, for example, a cystojejunal anastomosis, is to be carried out. Under sonographic control, puncture of the main pancreatic duct is not difficult, and a cyst is even less difficult to puncture. Finally, we must precisely define the vascular relations of the pancreas, in particular to the mesentericoportal venous axis, whose dissection is always difficult in exeresis for chronic pancreatitis.

5.5 Exocrine Pancreatic Cancer

Most cancers of the pancreas are ductular carcinomas. Macroscopically these appear as an indurated tumor of sclerotic consistency, which is why they have sometimes been called pancreatic scirrhus. The tumoral tissue is not homogeneous but consists of hemorrhagic foci and necrotic plaques. Furthermore, pancreatitis often occurs as a complication of cancer, mainly when the tumor is in the head (Fig. 5.17). This upstream pancreatitis is called epineoplastic pancreatitis. More seldom the cancer appears macroscopically as a soft friable mass with encephaloid features. This implies particularly significant tumoral necrosis [2].

This very brief review of macroscopic pathology explains the different sonographic aspects of exocrine pancreatic cancers. They appear as rounded tumors whose echogenicity is variable [8]. In the case of minimal necrosis but very dense sclerosis, the tumor is hyperechogenic. In contrast, in the presence of hemorrhage and necrotic foci, adenocarcinoma appears rather hypoechogenic. The more significant the necrosis, the less echogenic it is. In fact, notions of hypo- or hyperechogenicity are relative because the tissular echogenicity of these tumors is compared with the surrounding parenchyma which is often the seat of an associated reaction of pancreatitis that will be hyperechogenic. There is no pathognomonic sonographic criterion of pancreatic adenocarcinoma. Intraoperative sonography only allows confirmation of the diagnosis of a pancreatic mass. Thereafter, it helps

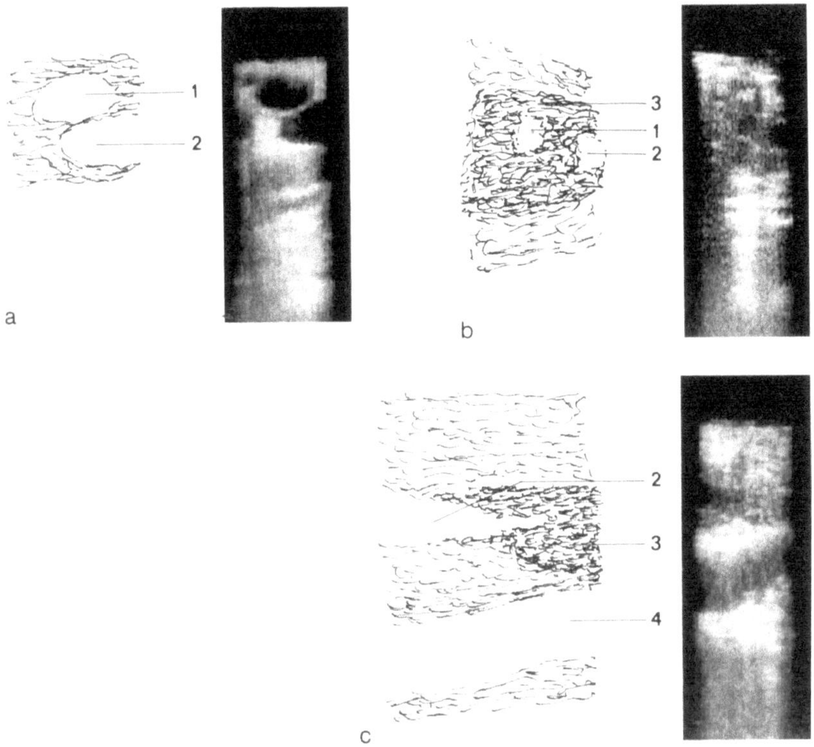

Fig. 5.17 a–c. Exocrine cancer of the head of pancreas. **a** Transverse section above the tumor: the bile duct is dilated, the portal vein is normal. **b** Transverse section through the superior pole of the tumor. The tumor encases the bile duct and the portal vein. **c** Longitudinal section of the portal vein with stenosis and invasion by tumor; *1*, common bile duct; *2*, portal vein; *3*, tumor; *4*, inferior vena cava

in effecting cytopunctures directed toward the tumoral center or in detecting indirect signs of pancreatic tumor. These indirect signs are bile duct stenosis or pancreatic duct stenosis, and upstream dilatation in the absence of lithiasis (Fig. 5.18). For us these findings are not of absolute value. However, intraoperative sonography is valuable in the diagnosis of vascular extension (Fig. 5.19). As a consequence of the richness of the vascular environment and its intimate relations to the gland, such extension is not rare. Initially, it occurs in the direction of the mesenterico-portal venous axis, then toward the superior mesenteric artery or the hepatic artery. Without sonography or ileoportography, only a long and delicate dissection enables verification of vascular involvement. Ileoportography is known as a long and invasive examination that is rarely practised during surgery. As well, celiomesenteric arteriography is not always included in intraoperative assessment. Finally, in practice the surgeon must begin to dissect earlier in order to know the extent of invasion of the peripancreatic vessels. Intraoperative sonography should enable us to know, before starting dissection, whether the vessels have been invaded or not, and whether vessels are to be sacrificed or not. It therefore permits rapid determi-

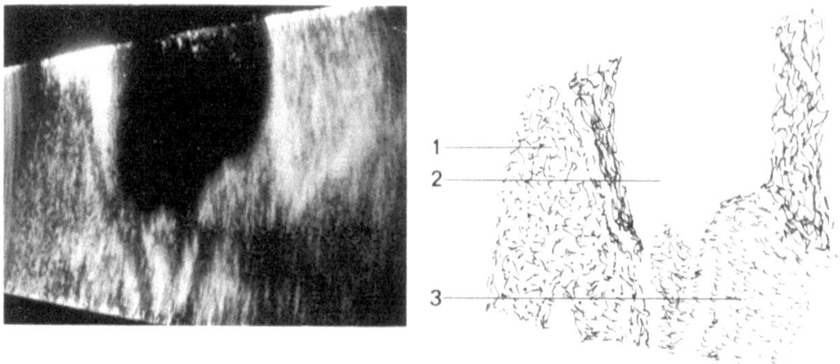

a

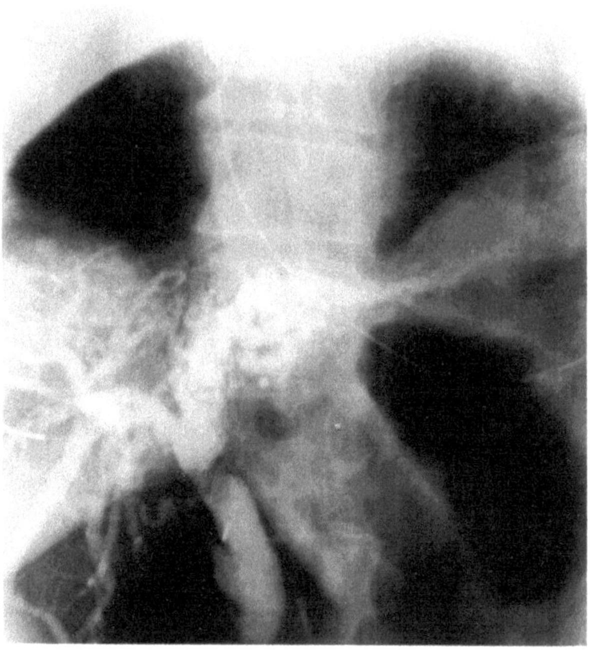

b

Fig. 5.18 a, b. Exocrine pancreatic cancer. **a** Intraoperative ultrasonography shows a small cephalic tumor invading the bile duct. Notice the hypoechogenic character of this tumor; *1*, duodenum; *2*, bile duct; *3*, tumor. **b** Intraoperative cholangiography allows additional discovery of a Caroli's disease in the left lobe of the liver

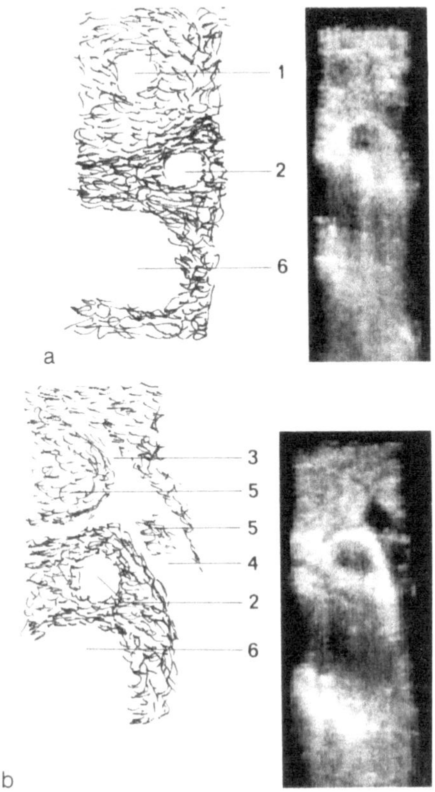

Fig. 5.19 a, b. Transverse sections showing pancreatic adenocarcinoma invading and thrombosing the mesentericoportal venous axis. **a** Portal vein invaded by tumor. The superior mesenteric artery is intact. **b** Section below the preceding one: there is neoplastic thrombus in the superior and inferior mesenteric veins; *1*, portal vein; *2*, superior mesenteric artery; *3*, superior mesenteric vein; *4*, inferior mesenteric vein; *5*, thrombus; *6*, aorta

nation of indications as well as operative technique. In short, in surgery for exocrine pancreatic cancer, intraoperative sonography can confirm the diagnosis of a pancreatic mass, provides information about contingent vascular extension, and permits the surgeon to search for occult hepatic metastasis.

5.6 Endocrine Tumors

Operative sonography may be used in several ways to assist the surgeon who is operating for endocrine tumor of the pancreas. The surgeon may find a nodule on the surface of the pancreas which may be suggestive of a tumor. In these situations, sonography can be used to confirm or exclude the possibility that the nodule actually is a tumor. Endocrine tumors are typically hypoechogenic. Thus, if a nodule presents such an appearance, the index of suspicion that a tumor is present must at once be raised. Conversely, if the nodule has the same echogenicity as the remainder of the gland, it is unlikely to be a tumor.

A more serious problem occurs if a pancreatic endocrine tumor cannot be palpated by the surgeon. In these situations a systematic scan of the gland with the ultrasound transducer may reveal tumors which would otherwise not be evident to the surgeon [7]. Such scanning is important in two different applications: firstly, systematic sonographic scanning of the pancreas is useful in detecting solitary tumors within the substance of the gland; secondly, comprehensive scanning of the pancreas should be performed after a solitary tumor has been detected and localized. The purpose of this maneuver is to ascertain whether multiple lesions are present.

Endocrine tumors anywhere in the body are almost always hypoechogenic relative to the surrounding tissue. This is particularly true of the pancreas with respect to the echogenic properties of surrounding pancreatic tissue, as shown in Figs. 5.20 and 5.21 [9]. The reason for such a decrease in echogenicity probably relates to the homogeneous structure of such tumors and the minimal presence of boundary layers produced by stromal elements which would cause an increase in reflectivity. The hypoechogenic nature of endocrine tumors is a fortuitous property, in that it greatly facilitates the use of ultrasound for their detection.

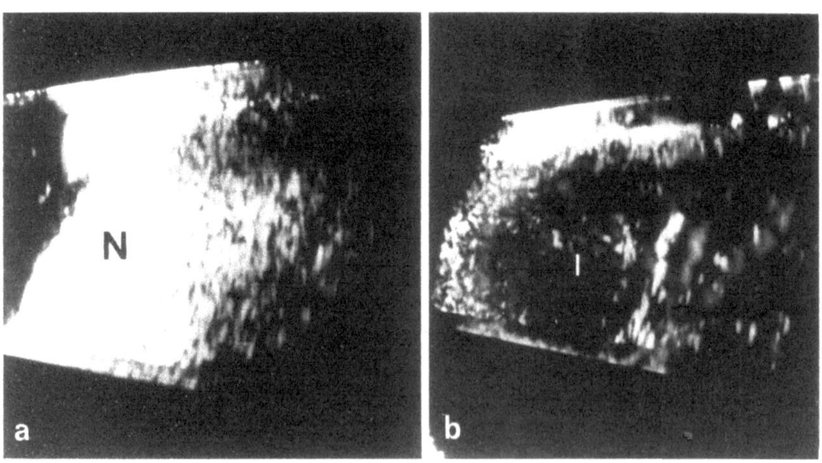

Fig. 5.20 a, b. Composite of two sonograms obtained from the same pancreas. **a** Normal pancreatic tissue (*N*). **b** Insulinoma (*I*) with a covering rim of normal pancreas. The insulinoma is less echogenic than the normal pancreas

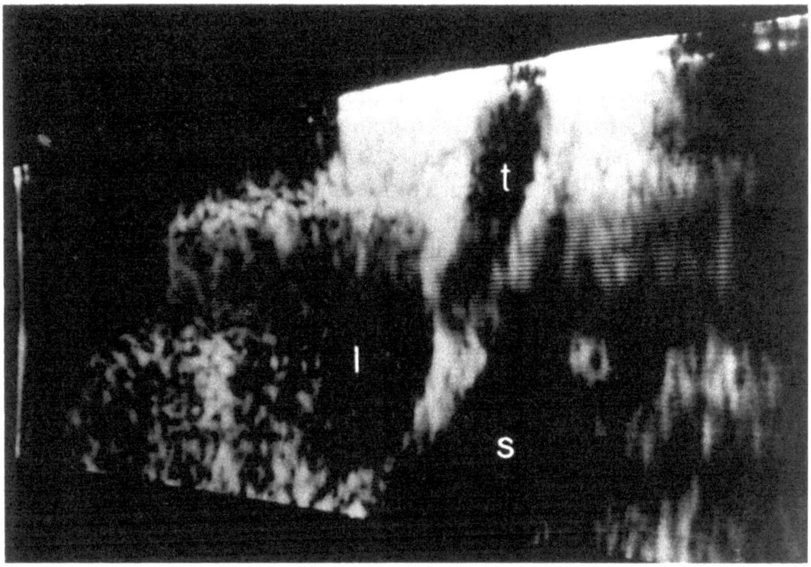

Fig. 5.21. Pancreatic sonogram shows a sonolucent structure which proved to be an insulinoma (*I*). The splenic vein (*S*) and a tributary vein (*t*) are seen deep to the insulinoma

The problems of a false-negative examination are principally related to the size of the lesion. The smallest lesions that we have detected were 4 mm in diameter. It is possible that ultrasound will miss lesions which are below this size. There are several causes of false-positive examinations. One is the visualization of a hypoechogenic area which is caused by conditions other than an endocrine tumor. The main causes of such a finding are tissue spaces, veins, ducts and lymph nodes. Tissue spaces are usually irregular, in contrast to the smooth, rounded appearance of tumors. Veins may demonstrate moving luminal echoes. Veins and ducts appear as rounded structures in cross-section, but when the transducer is turned through 90°, they appear elongated. Lymph nodes are probably the most difficult structures to differentiate from endocrine tumors. They are usually superficial to the gland and may have to be biopsied in order to make a final confirmation of their nature.

5.7 Discussion

From a general point of view, the sonographic features of certain lesions, their topography, vascular and ductural relations, and the precise guidance of puncture needles are several elements contributing to diagnosis and choice of the most appropriate surgical procedure.

5.7.1 Chronic Pancreatitis

It is easy to rapidly assess the volume and parenchymatous structure of the gland, to see calcifications, and to verify from the image the predominant involvement of the right or left pancreas. The pancreatic parenchyma appears heterogeneous and hyperechogenic. Calcifications are represented by many very echogenic points. If the latter are numerous enough, interpretation of the image is hampered. The main pancreatic duct is easily detectable, its caliber often being greater than normal. Its puncture by needle becomes very easy, as do sampling pancreatic juice and carrying out opacification. Exact determination of its caliber, evidence of irregularities, associated cysts, and intraductular lithiases rapidly yield important information that is useful for the choice of internal bypass or exeresis.

Concerning pancreatic pseudocysts, the information provided by sonography is also interesting, as there is no problem in determining the cyst's volume, its relations to adjacent organs, or in checking the appearance of the remaining pancreas. Assuming as a hypothesis the need for internal bypass, it is advisable to first define the thickness of the wall in order to perform the cystoenteric anastomosis under optimal conditions.

Is intraoperative sonography sufficient for perfect investigation of chronic pancreatitis? The answer has to be full of nuances. In practice, sonography has become a basic examination for the reasons just mentioned. However, we still carry out pancreatography, and/or cholangiography, if we judge it useful. Only radiologic opacification provides a dynamic view of the passage of the contrast medium into the duodenum. In the same way, very often only opacification permits objective assessment of the communication of a cyst with the main pancreatic duct. Under certain circumstances, when the information from the sonographic examination seems insufficient, we cannot do without the data furnished by radiology. There is, however, no doubt that intraoperative sonography is an essential examination, because independently it enabled us in a large series to modify the operative technique in 60% of cases [9].

5.7.2 Exocrine Pancreatic Cancers

Too often nowadays, intraoperative examination can only assert the diagnosis of a pancreatic mass and not formally establish its malignant nature. Consequently, intraoperative exploration has to confirm the diagnosis of cancer and determine its local and regional extension. What role does sonography play here?

In the diagnosis of adenocarcinoma of the exocrine pancreas, ultrasonography has limited advantages. Of course, it confirms the diagnosis of a pancreatic mass, but there are no sonographic criteria with which these cancers can be assessed. Their echogenicity can be less than, equal to, or greater than that of the surrounding pancreatic tissue, which itself can be normal or the seat of pancreatitis [8]. The sonographic appearance of a pancreatic mass precludes any judgment about its nature, no image being specific to, or characteristic of, adenocarcinoma. In spite of the absence of sonographic signs (the mass itself being the only sign), there are indirect signs of some value: stenosis of the bile duct or main pancreatic duct, upstream dilatation of ducts, and the absence of lithiasis. Finally, sonography can help in directing cytopunctures toward the center of the mass.

When a diagnosis of adenocarcinoma has been formally established by the pathologist, its extent must be determined exactly, so as to be able to make a choice between curative exeresis and palliative surgery. Sonography can be very useful here. In fact, two types of extension, among others, can lead to renouncement of exeresis, if not detected during preoperative investigation: invasion of peripancreatic vessels and the presence of hepatic metastasis.

Concerning vascular examination, sonography allows good visualization of the mesentericoportal venous axis and the superior mesenteric and hepatic arteries. As a consequence, the surgeon knows quickly, before starting dissection, whether vascular sacrifices will be necessary or not.

Referring to hepatic metastasis, the possibility of sonographic detection of subclinical metastases has already been mentioned (see Chapter 3). Sonographic exploration has a lot to teach us about adenocarcinoma. In practice it is sufficient as an intraoperative technique of imagery. Radiology cannot be considered complementary. Cholangiography and pancreatography are of little advantage, and ileoportography, being a cumbersome and invasive examination, is not justified anymore.

5.7.3 Endocrine Pancreatic Tumors

The difficulties encountered in localizing certain endocrine tumors of the pancreas are known. The principal obstacle is the usually small size (often less than 15 mm) of the most common types: insulomas and gastrinomas. Sonography, computed tomography, arteriography and sequential elevations of hormone levels within the pancreatic and peripancreatic veins give us the opportunity to localize the majority of tumors before intervention. Nevertheless, 20%-25% of insulomas [10, 11], and 26%-50% of gastrinomas [3, 5] are not found again upon surgical exploration. With respect to the latter, the frequency of multifocal lesions makes the problem even more complex.

Endocrine pancreatic tumors are sufficiently characteristic to be identified by sonography. They appear rounded, hypoechogenic in comparison to the surrounding pancreatic tissue, and are quite well demarcated [4, 9]. Sonographic exploration must be thorough, without neglecting any sector of the pancreas, in order to avoid overlooking multifocal forms. The fact is, however, that it has its limits, particularly in diffuse forms of gastrinoma, in which some adenomatous foci are smaller than 3 mm, and cannot be detected [8]. Likewise, in certain diffuse hyperplasias, an attempt at morphologic investigation of an individual tumor focus is hopeless. Fortunately, these cases are rare, and most of the time intraoperative sonography is very helpful. It can confirm the site of a tumor discovered by preoperative investigation, the endocrine tumoral nature of a small mass palpated by the surgeon and, finally, detect other lesions that were not perceptible during either preoperative examination or laparotomy. As a consequence, it reduces surgical exploration time and avoids futile capsulotomies.

5.7.4 Acute Pancreatitis

We have no experience with intraoperative sonography in acute pancreatitis. Nonetheless, it has been used successfully in searching for sequestra or a residual abscess [1]. It can actually be very helpful in following up acute pancreatitis in patients who have undergone single, or sometimes multiple, surgical intervention. Collections of inflammatory exudate have the sonographic appearance of abscesses and are generally represented by anechogenic zones occupied by echoes that correspond to necrotic fragments.

References

1. Alexandre JH, Hernigou A, Billebaud T, Bouillot JL, Plainfosse MC (1985) Echotomographie per-opératoire du pancréas. Gastroenterol Clin Biol 9: 572-577
2. Baumel H, Deixonne B (1986) Pancreatic exocrine cancer. Springer-Verlag, Berlin Heidelberg New York Tokyo
3. Bonfils S, Landor JH, Mignon M, Hervoir P (1981) Results of surgical management in 92 consecutive patients with Zollinger-Ellison syndrome. Ann Surg 194: 692-697
4. Chapuis Y, Hernigou A, Plainfosse MC, Bonnette P (1984) Exemples d'application de l'ultrasonographie - temps réel per-opératoire en chirurgie endocrinienne. Chirurgie 110: 97-104
5. Deveney CW, Deveney KS, Way LW (1978) The Zollinger-Ellison syndrome, 23 years later. Ann Surg 188: 384-391
6. Mercadier M (1985) Management of chronic pancreatitis. In: Advances in hepatic, biliary and pancreatic surgery, 1979-1986. Year Book Medical Publishers, Chicago, USA
7. Norton J, Sigel B, Baker A et al (1985) Localization of an occult insulinoma by intra-operative ultrasonography. Surgery 97: 381-384
8. Sigel B, Coelho JC, Nyhus LM et al (1982) Detection of pancreatic tumors by ultrasound during surgery. Arch Surg 117: 1058-1061
9. Sigel B, Duarte B, Coelho JC et al (1983) Localization of insulinomas of the pancreas at operation by real-time ultrasound scanning. Surg Gynaecol Obstet 156: 145-147
10. Stefanini P, Carboni M, Patrassi N, Basoli A (1974) Beta-islet tumors of the pancreas: results of a study on 1067 cases. Surgery 75: 597-609
11. Xianju Z, Yu Z, Weiran W, Tonghua L (1980) Insulinoma diagnostic and therapeutic experiences in 60 cases. Clin Med J 93: 149-158

6 Subject Index

MIX
Papier aus verantwortungsvollen Quellen
Paper from responsible sources
FSC® C105338

If you have any concerns about our products,
you can contact us on
ProductSafety@springernature.com

In case Publisher is established outside the EU,
the EU authorized representative is:
Springer Nature Customer Service Center GmbH
Europaplatz 3, 69115 Heidelberg, Germany

Printed by Libri Plureos GmbH
in Hamburg, Germany